The Fourth Trimester

The publisher gratefully acknowledges the generous support of Jamie Rosenthal Wolf, David Wolf, Rick Rosenthal, and Nancy Stephens as members of the Publisher's Circle of the University of California Press Foundation.

The publisher also gratefully acknowledges the generous support of the General Endowment Fund of the University of California Press Foundation.

The Fourth Trimester

*Understanding, Protecting, and
Nurturing an Infant through
the First Three Months*

Susan Brink

UNIVERSITY OF CALIFORNIA PRESS
Berkeley   Los Angeles   London

University of California Press, one of the most distinguished university presses in the United States, enriches lives around the world by advancing scholarship in the humanities, social sciences, and natural sciences. Its activities are supported by the UC Press Foundation and by philanthropic contributions from individuals and institutions. For more information, visit www.ucpress.edu.

University of California Press
Berkeley and Los Angeles, California

University of California Press, Ltd.
London, England

Library of Congress Cataloging-in-Publication Data

Brink, Susan (Susan Frances)
    The fourth trimester : understanding, protecting, and nurturing an infant through the first three months / Susan Brink.
        p.   cm.
    Includes bibliographical references and index.
    ISBN 978-0-520-26712-1 (cloth : alk. paper)
    1. Infants—Development.   2. Infants—Care.   3. Newborn infants—Development.   4. Newborn infants—Care.   I. Title.
    HQ774.B755   2013
    649'.122—dc23   2012013037

Manufactured in the United States of America

20 19 18 17 16 15 14 13
10 9 8 7 6 5 4 3 2 1

In keeping with a commitment to support environmentally responsible and sustainable printing practices, UC Press has printed this book on Rolland Enviro100, a 100% postconsumer fiber paper that is FSC certified, deinked, processed chlorine-free, and manufactured with renewable biogas energy. It is acid-free and EcoLogo certified.

To Max, Makayla, Maggie, Ariana, Carissa,
and Molly
And in loving memory of Nancy

CONTENTS

PREFACE

My commitment to write a book about the newborn's first three months comes from my own life. I married very young and have two daughters and six grandchildren. Yet nothing from my maternal experience or from my professional background as a journalist specializing in science and medicine eased me or my grown children through the sudden shock of being completely responsible for the life and development of a brand-new human being.

On my desk I have photographs that tell the story. The snapshots I took a few days before my daughters became mothers show them proudly posing with their full-term pregnant bodies in profile, their smiles broad and genuine. Then comes a shot of my daughter Jenny, triumphant with her newborn Max, but her smile has become uncertain. The same uncertainty is written on Rachel's face in yet another snapshot, her eyes wary and full of doubt, posing with one-day-old Makayla. As brand-new mothers, my daughters had had their confidence seriously shaken.

I look at those photographs and recall my own shock decades ago when nurses handed over my firstborn. How could they be so reckless as to entrust a helpless new human being to clueless me?

We all made it through, my daughters and I, as new parents do. Yet I know that for the first three months we relied on trial and error, intuition, dumb luck—and the passing of time.

Three months, said pediatricians, other mothers, friends, and family. Just hang in there for three months, and the mysterious and demanding infant will become more human, more like the baby you imagined. Since embarking on the research for this book, I understand in a deeper way why, during the fourth trimester of development, an infant is not like the baby that people imagine. I want others to be able to do more than just hang in there while they anxiously wait for three months to pass. This book is for parents, grandparents, friends, family members, physicians, and students, every single one of them eager to do the right thing by each infant he or she encounters. I want everyone who is in awe of and in love with a newborn to understand exactly how to protect and nurture an infant during the first three months of life—the critically important fourth trimester.

Susan Brink

Introduction

*A Transition from the Comfort of the Womb
to the Reality of the World*

Like parents everywhere, David and Tammy DiGregorio were under the illusion that they were ready for the arrival of their firstborn child. They knew she was a girl and that they would name her Ava. The West Hollywood parents had carefully gathered an extensive array of newborn equipment, read the recommended books, taken Lamaze classes, practiced panting and breathing for her birth, and attended newborn classes offered by their hospital. And sure enough, the birth, delivery, and hospital stay went off without a hitch.

Then they brought Ava home, and all anxiety broke loose. "I was terrified," says Tammy. "I was handed this little baby, and it was a complete shock. I was so tired and so scared; I felt like I was in a whole other world," she continues. "And I was terrified of making a mistake." As for baby Ava, well . . . "She was like a strange little alien."[1]

Such is the coming-home of many, alas most, newborns who are long awaited and eagerly welcomed. Before women even have time to complete a full sigh of relief signaling the end to forty weeks of awkward discomfort, they find themselves facing even greater challenges. Only now, with actual infants in their arms, they have far less control. Ava, like any newborn, was barely equipped to stay alive. Tammy and David were suddenly face to face with the most neurologically immature of all the earth's primates, born months before she was anywhere near ready to function in the world.

Parents around the world who welcome mysterious new life in this way encounter a significant void in up-to-date scientific information about the first days and weeks of infancy. With fingers crossed, they confront their uncertainty and fears.

This book presents a new paradigm of a baby's early life that shifts our focus and alters our priorities. It shows that this window of time, specifically the first three months of life, has more in common with what came before than with what follows. The fourth trimester is an outside-the-uterus period of intense development that is an extension of the work begun during the first nine months. A newborn human is not so much a baby as a final-phase fetus living through a time of transition as he gives up the comforts of the uterus and gradually adjusts to the wonders and challenges of the world. Further, during this period infants and mothers need to stay almost as tightly bound together as biology dictated during the first three trimesters. In this book, I use the model of a fourth trimester to show how parents, caregivers, doctors, and students might understand this period by looking at it through a new lens.

Throughout, I talk about the essential bond between a loving, committed, and attentive adult and a baby. Sometimes that attachment is biologically unique to birth mother and baby. Born recognizing her voice and her smell and, for most of human evolution, dependent on her milk, an infant bonds most quickly with his mother.

But in our complex and ever-changing society, it's important to think broadly and not give short shrift to any woman or man who "mothers" an infant. An adoptive parent—mother, father, married, single, gay, or straight—can read references to "mother" and "father" in these pages and know it speaks to them just as it does to biological parents. Be assured, this is not simply lip service. Though biology counts for a lot in favoring birth mothers, the book's importance to fathers and nonbiological parents represents more than an artifact of the past few decades of a changing culture. The bond between parents and non-biological offspring represents an evolutionary moral and medical breakthrough on parenting that no doubt is being, and will increasingly be, studied over generations.

Within this book, the advice and much of the science can apply to all who give birth to or adopt babies, as well as to those who watch over, nourish, nurture, and protect an infant in the first hours and days of life. Under that wide umbrella, I mean to give respectful due to all kinds of parents—birth mothers and fathers, adoptive parents, same-sex partners, single parents, grandmothers, grandfathers, and all manner of kith and kin. Any one person or pair or team of people responsible for the nurturance, care, and protection of a newborn is fully able to provide, and can be equally expert in providing, the love, diligence, and attention that every baby needs.

Infants are nothing if not flexible, ready to respond to love. Here's an analogy. I had a cat once, a calico, that loved me best. She curled up on my lap. She slept in my bed. She was as cozy with me as a cat can be. But once, she disappeared from the house for a few days. I put up posters, and soon a man was at my door holding my Irma. What surprised me was how quickly she had switched allegiance. She was curled up in this stranger's arms as though he were the love of her life. I almost hated to separate them as he handed her back to me.

This is not just the sentimental musing of a pet lover. Certainly, newborns are a lot more complicated, but in some ways they're a bit like my fickle cat. An infant will love the one she's with. And long before she can show love, she will respond to the one she's with. He can be fed with a tender touch, with locked-in eye contact from a birth father or mother. She can have her diaper changed to the accompaniment of chipper conversation by an adoptive parent and, in the blink of an eye, will recognize his voice above all others even though she didn't hear it in the womb. He can listen as a same-sex couple sings a lullaby duet. The mother who supplied the egg responsible for half his genetic makeup—but whose uterus did not house him— can soothe him. The father who devotes himself to the baby, regardless of whose sperm fertilized the egg all those months ago, can rock her to sleep. Newborns will thrive even as the definition of *family* changes to incorporate not only traditional marriages and adoptive parents but also gay marriages, single-parent families, combined families, grandparents raising second generations of children, and as many configurations as loving people can come up with to create the protective, nurturing nest that is a family.

Combining contemporary science with the personal stories of dozens of parents I interviewed—as well as a few of my own—I've attempted to write to all who nurture. Science has a lot to say to each and every one of them about the hows and whys of caring for a newborn. The word *caretaker* or *caregiver* is hardly sufficient to describe a person who changes diapers, is at the ready at all hours, sings, soothes, tries to project a calm front despite his own worry, plays, feeds, rocks, cradles, and would throw himself under a bus to protect a newborn. But *loving care-taker* and *caregiver* are convenient shorthand terms I sometimes use. Know that these are written with profound respect for all the people who love and tend to every need of a newborn throughout the fourth trimester.

The infant, amazingly competent yet totally dependent, needs all of them. The nine-month gestation prepared the fetus well, but incompletely. A newborn can hear, but cannot sort through the din. He can discern light, shadow, and contrast, but cannot "see" as we understand vision. She can feel, but the womb provided protection and warmth that she continues to need postpartum. In the uterus, taste and smell filtered through amniotic fluid, making him recognize the odor of colostrum and the taste of mother's milk. The newborn is prepared to begin learning the new world she's entered, but this period, which is closely linked to fetal life and is beginning to prepare her for real life, is one of transition during which she needs close, constant, and loving attention.

This book is primarily intended for new parents and care-givers who want more than to be told how to care for a new-born. They want to understand the reasons behind the advice. It will also be useful to anyone called upon to give guidance (doctors, nurses, teachers) and to those with a personal interest in understanding the well-being of a newborn (friends, relatives, grandparents). Each chapter of this book translates the most current science in a specific area of early infant development into a rationale for appropriate care. In a field where opinion and trendy advice are seldom connected to evidence, this book presents a clear and much-needed alternative.

Journalism skills, honed over a thirty-year career in medical reporting, helped me to arrive at this reasoned and evidence-based alternative. Journalists are adept at following all leads while pursuing a range of sources. They get an overview of an issue—not merely the pediatrician's view from the clinic, the scientist's view from the lab, the parent's view from the nursery, or the investigator's view from reading the latest research. The knowledge and wisdom of all those players inform the chapters, synthesized and interpreted for the curious new parents and caregivers eager for this information.

A report by the National Research Council and Institute of Medicine on children and brain development, published in 2000, became my starting point. The report's conclusions have rippled through every aspect of science, medicine, and education and into family homes. This report, *From Neurons to Neighborhoods: The Science of Early Childhood Development,* says, "Although there have been long-standing debates about how much the early years really matter in the larger scheme of lifelong development, our conclusion is unequivocal: What happens during the first months and years of life matters a lot, not because this period of development provides an indelible blueprint for adult well-being, but because it sets either a sturdy or fragile stage for what follows."[2]

Readers will appreciate the distinction. Adhering to the best that science has to recommend during the fourth trimester does not present an "indelible blueprint," since infants, babies, and children can and do overcome poor beginnings. But why start them out by giving them a lot to overcome? Rather, let's do our best to set the stage for "sturdy" development by treating the first three months of life as the biological continuation of fetal development that it is.

New research has begun to change thinking, establishing the fourth trimester as an especially vital time for laying down the very foundations of development. Yet this excellent science is not without controversy, as currently interpreted by the popular media and various advocacy groups. Two particularly inflamed hot-button issues are breast feeding versus formula feeding and cosleeping versus sleeping alone. Acknowledging a variety of opinions on these issues, the text sticks to the research while recognizing that science is a leading factor, but not the *only* factor, in parents' decisions on feeding and sleeping arrangements. In this objective way, the book stands apart in providing a comprehensive survey of a newborn's developmental needs while remaining intimate, personal, and nonjudgmental. It can help new parents—biological or adoptive, as well as others who provide consistent love and attention to infants— make their own personal decisions within the parameters of best practices.

The need for loving attention is a constant theme of this book. Each chapter also draws on personal interviews with prominent researchers, practitioners, and parents. These resources are documented in the text in sufficient detail for a curious reader to pursue specific questions in the relevant literature.

The first three months of an infant's life need not be a mystery to bumble through. It's a common joke that infants don't come with an operating manual. This compilation of recent medical, biological, neurological, behavioral, developmental, and social science research from the past two decades provides the basis for just such an operating manual. New parents can comprehend much of what throughout human history has been inexplicable and, in the process, get their babies off to the best possible start.

The book begins millions of years ago with the chapter "Evolution and the Primitive Brain of a Newborn." It is the natural starting point in helping parents and caretakers understand that the reason human infants arrive so unfinished is deeply rooted in our common evolution—beginning with the moment our hominid ancestors first stood and walked on two legs. Readers will understand why forty weeks of gestation is both a biological imperative and insufficient for greater brain development in the uterus. They will begin to see that all newborns need another three months, a fourth trimester, of uncompromisingly close connection to their mothers or an equally loving and attentive caretaker.

The remainder of the book is organized by first addressing how such an immature brain influences infants' most basic needs: crying, sleeping, and eating. These behaviors deserve three distinct chapters since they are the source of every parent's most urgent worries. These three concerns are linked to each other just as communication is linked to need. Every newborn cry of life reminds us that this human being isn't ready to be separated from the uterus. Food, warmth, soothing movement, and comfort once flowed to her without effort. Now, she must signal hunger, discomfort, and fear with a cry, at first her only tool of communication. Now, as she makes her transition from the womb to the world, each adult response to her wailing demands is helping to complete the neurological wiring vital for living. The comforting closeness so recently experienced by the fetus continues as chemicals released by physical contact or close proximity to a mother, father, or caring adult help the newborn regulate sleep and arousal.[3] Food, passively received in the womb, now requires effort.

The best nutritional transition to the real world during the fourth trimester, as evolution and biology make clear, is breast milk. A clear understanding that breast feeding is the most natural extension of pregnancy is an important starting point for every birth mother as she makes her own decision. I balance that truth with the reality that some women cannot breast-feed or don't want to. Adoptive parents, foster parents, grandparents, and all manner of attentive caretakers cannot breast-feed. For them, formula is a perfectly adequate second-best choice as they, too, help their newborn with the transition to life in the world by holding the infant closely, making eye contact, and touching him. What he has received without asking for during nine months in the uterus—food, soothing comfort, sleeping on his own timetable—must continue during the time of transition via attentive response to his cries.

Even as the basic needs for soothing, sleep, and food are met, the senses are proving to be nature's first teachers. After addressing parents' most urgent concerns, the book's next chapters delve deeply into sensory development—sound, sight, and touch. (Taste and smell, scientifically studied in far less depth in newborns and tightly linked to feeding, are discussed in the feeding chapter.) Nothing in infant development happens in isolation, and these three senses are intimately connected to soothing, sleeping, and eating. But these senses each deserve a closer look. Babies recognize their mothers' voices at the moment of birth because they've heard them in the uterus. Hearing these voices again during the fourth trimester is an important part of the transition, and newborns turn to their mothers' voices more readily than to any others. (Though, in the case of adoptive parents or alternative caretakers, babies will soon recognize a consistent new voice and will turn to the voice they've come to know.) From the moment of birth, infants are busy soaking up the acoustics of their surroundings.

Vision is less developed than hearing at birth, but newborns can already see shadows of eyes, edges of faces, and areas of high contrast. Newborns see better than once thought, but the concept of "seeing" is complex, since vision consists of multiple components—focus, contrast, three-dimensionality, color—all developing at varying rates. Furthermore, the areas of the brain that interpret what's coming through the eyes are not yet set up to register what's seen in the way adults understand vision. Yet astonishingly, the very act of seeing is exactly what babies need in order to sort it all out. Each flicker of vision is setting up neural connections that will eventually let babies see the full world around them. The relatively slowly developing sense of vision carries infants forward from a place of darkness in the womb into a world of light.

The sense of touch, influenced for forty weeks by the warmth of amniotic fluid and the secure confines of the uterus, continues during this time of transition through swaddling, cuddling, and stroking. The last fifteen years have seen a sea change in understanding touch, both painful and pleasurable types. Simple, human touch—comforting pats in response to tears, smiles in response to contented moments—releases brain chemicals that calm the infant. On the other hand, trauma and stress (abuse, neglect, pain) release a flood of neurochemicals, including cortisol, that can set a child up for future trouble.

There are coexisting truths about the development of the senses: infants come into the world highly immature and yet extremely capable of learning and communicating. Each sense, at its own stage of readiness at birth, interacts with all the others to mold a brain that is forming the likes, dislikes, and very personality of a new human being.

As the senses are developing brand-new connections in the brain, the body is growing stronger. Neurological and physical developments are linked—these are similar to the mind-body connections science now recognizes in adults. Just as every interaction with the senses is building better abilities to see, hear, and feel, every kick is building muscles that will soon enable the baby to crawl, walk, and run. Biological mothers know that these early flailings begin during gestation, and many fathers have felt their force as they've laid a hand on a pregnant belly. An important chapter on physical development shows why the "exercise" begun in the womb must continue, with caretakers encouraging infants to vary their positions during awake time. Holding infants in various positions not only strengthens muscles, but it also gives infants a view of the world from more than one perspective, each view affecting the synapses being formed.

Almost universally, parents, regardless of their circumstances or limitations, want to do the best for their children. But with conflicting advice from the media, and with an array of books and toys promising smart and happy infants, parents can be confused about what course to follow. To put their minds at ease, a chapter on stimulation summarizes appropriate sensory stimulation. Loving attention to cries, along with soothing voices, comforting touches, eye contact, and closeness to the mother's body (or an equally loving caretaker's body) are the kinds of stimulation an infant needs. A view of a mother's face, a father's profile, the sound of live voices, the touch of skin or flannel or tweed, the smells of healthy foods cooking, and the taste of milk are preparing infants for the inimitable world that envelops them. For millions of years, trees, grass, voices, music, cuddling, constant proximity to mothers, and loving human interaction have provided all the stimulation infants need.

Finally, the book steps away from the newborn to delve into research on parents. Physical and psychological studies examining the postpartum months as experienced by mothers are extensive, and there are exciting new indications that, just as human interaction is sculpting infant brains, those same interactions are reshaping maternal brains. Research into fathers' health is fledgling, but science now knows that men, too, are susceptible to postpartum depression and that welcoming a child into a family can be stressful for both parents.

The multiple lines of research upon which this book is based show that a well-equipped brain is grown from the normal, simple, and readily available seeds of playful activity and loving parents and adults. The chatter of everyday life, lullabies of love, and glimpses of blue sky through green branches surrounding a newborn are naturally programming language, art, music, math, dexterity on the playground, and lifelong social skills.

This book will help put to rest the remnants of a century of cultural misconceptions that still linger: infant independence, fixed IQ, and a substitution of quality time for quantity time.

Cultural norms, fading but not entirely gone, once encouraged parents to make their largely unformed infants partly independent from day one. Infants were expected to go it alone in their own rooms, to figure out how to soothe themselves by crying themselves to sleep, to wait through hunger pangs for an appointed feeding hour—or to eat more than they wanted, which, the parents could hope, would then cause them to sleep longer. About a hundred years ago, this approach was encouraged by "male physicians who not only had never changed a diaper, but had never—in any substantial way—associated with, or taken care of their own infants," according to Dr. James Mc-Kenna, director of the Mother-Baby Behavioral Sleep Laboratory at the University of Notre Dame.[4] Separating infants from their parents was supposed to foster independent toddlers, children, and adults, and this approach was practiced for decades. Current research shows that it has the opposite effect.

The mid–twentieth century was also a time when people believed intelligence was fixed, set in stone at birth. In the 1950s and 1960s, research began to cast doubt on that assumption. We now know that a child's IQ is influenced greatly by either environmental stimulation or environmental neglect.[5] Science now sees the human brain in a kind of computer model: hardware delivered at birth, and software continually programmed by experience. The programming begins at birth at a breathtaking pace.

The 1970s introduced to popular culture the concept of "quality time." Parents could be absent for long stretches of their infants' days, the reasoning went, as long as they compensated for lost time by making every available moment of togetherness count with joyful, stimulating interaction. The trouble is, brain development doesn't take time off, and infants don't learn on a convenient schedule. When it comes to time, infants need both quality and sheer quantity. There are no shortcuts. A parent or a consistent, loving caretaker must be there when infants need them. During the fourth trimester, that's all the time.

This book goes a long way in removing the cloak of mystery that has always surrounded the fourth trimester. It presents an original perspective on the period following birth, identifying it as a continuation of the period of development within the uterus and, simultaneously, an interval that helps infants make the transition to the world.

This fresh way for parents, educators, and health care workers to understand newborns points to a difficult societal dilemma. Newborns require constant loving attention. That is a truth that must not be compromised by simple ignorance. Evolution and biology clearly prefer the bond to be between the newborn and the mother, though, as I've noted, infants can be well cared for by fathers, adoptive mothers and fathers, or other consistent, loving, attentive adults. This book points to the need to pay attention to infants twenty-four hours a day throughout the fourth trimester. Coming up with policy solutions that are truly family centered is beyond the scope of this book. But as a society, we need to come up with ways—*paid* parental leave for biological and adoptive mothers or fathers or both, for example—to support young families by ensuring that every infant is able to spend this crucial period of development held tightly in the arms of love.

CHAPTER ONE

Evolution and the Primitive Brain of a Newborn

Why Infants Arrive Unfinished

Blame Lucy. In the throes of labor contractions and delivery, remember that it was this 3.2-million-year-old human ancestor who first had the big idea to stand up and walk on two feet. Lucy is considered by many scientists to be the mother of humankind, and her skeletal remains, discovered in 1974, provided scientific evidence of one of the first upright walkers in our family tree.[1] From that point onward, the human ability to walk on two feet would demand some reworking of the adult pelvis and a major overhaul of the birth canal. Those evolving alterations would, in all descendant female hominids leading up to *Homo sapiens,* introduce a host of inefficient twists and turns, making the process long and painful for mothers and a brutal challenge for babies.

Lucy's hypothetical offspring, no longer able to survive with the limited brainpower required to climb a tree or flee from danger on four legs, needed more time to grow a bigger brain in order to outwit predators. But a maximum of forty weeks' gestation is all that biology allowed our ancient

ancestors and modern babies. They would need a fourth trimester of intense development experienced outside the uterus
while remaining physically and emotionally bound to their
mothers, just as they had been for the previous nine months.
The tight fit through that circuitous birth canal set abso-
lute limits on how much brain development could occur during pregnancy. The additional brain growth required to keep
the species thriving would have to happen outside the
uterus, an astonishing amount of it occurring during the
fourth trimester.

Modern human infants are at the receiving end of millions
of years of evolutionary progress, but the tradeoff for upright
walking has been immature brain development at birth.

Walking on two feet has been a mixed blessing. Standing
upright altered the entire skeletal structure, and the changes
came with physical costs for males and females: flat feet, ach-
ing backs, and stiff necks. "Ultimately, every part of the human
body had to change to adapt to bipedalism," says Dr. Wenda
Trevathan, evolutionary anthropologist at the University of
New Mexico.[2]

Women and infants have suffered especially onerous consequences of upright posture. What was once a straight shot down
a roomy birth canal in our four-legged ancestors has evolved
into something akin to an amusement park ride through the
modern female pelvis.

Once humans had only two feet for mobility, they could no
longer climb as well as, or run as fast as, the local lions and
tigers and bears. Since then, they've had to rely on brainpower
to escape predators. The pressure for increased intelligence was
on, and our ancient forebears began to grow brains far larger
than ever before. In fact, the human brain *had* to get bigger, or

our species would have died out. Those outsized brains, and resulting intelligence, began to change the world.

As the human brain has grown in size during evolution, the additional brain growth needed for survival has had to take place after birth because there simply is no extra room in the birth canal for a bigger head.[3] After roughly nine months in the uterus, emerge babies must, ready or not. Most aspects of brain development are delayed until after birth. "And that means the baby is a little more *unfinished,* if you will," says Dr. Trevathan. "The evolutionary compromise is that about 75 percent of human brain development takes place after birth." That's in contrast with the rest of the animal kingdom. Most animals are born with their brains about half developed, but today human infants are born with only 26 percent to 29 percent of their brains developed. And so, with a brain only about a quarter of its necessary size, the newborn needs a fourth trimester of development, with comforts similar to those enjoyed in the womb preparing him for life in the world.

THE BIRTH RIDE

The evolutionary compromise between the need for a large brain and the confines of a narrow birth canal continues with modern-day infants. They arrive extremely neurologically immature and completely dependent on adults.

Leading, in most cases, with a head that can accommodate roughly a quarter of the brain mass she'll eventually require, the fetus is forced to negotiate a series of turns aligned with the widest parts of the pelvis. The entrance of the birth canal is widest from side to side. About halfway through, the orientation shifts about ninety degrees, and the fetus must turn her large head to make it through. So the infant starts her journey facing her mother's side. Midway she must shift her head to face her mother's back. As the fetus's head turns from facing her mother's side to facing her back, she goes through a series of rotations as she passes through the birth canal. Once the head has emerged, the shoulders must shift, so the baby turns her head to the side, rotating her shoulders so they, too, can make the tight squeeze between pubic bones and tailbone.[4]

The average infant head is ten centimeters from front to back. It's little wonder that childbirth hurts, considering that the average woman's pelvic opening is thirteen centimeters at its largest point and ten centimeters at its smallest point.

The quadruped ancestors of modern humans, with larger birth canals and smaller brains, once might have given birth in solitude—like chimpanzees, orangutans, and gorillas can. However, because of the revised size and position of the human female pelvis, women need midwifelike assistance to give birth. If the mother reached down to assist her own baby's birth, she would risk injuring her baby by bending his back against the natural curve of the spine.

As a result, not only did human bodies change with upright walking, but society also had to change in ways that could accommodate the demands placed on the mother by the baby. First, mothers couldn't deliver in solitude. Once here, babies could not cling with hands and feet, so mothers had to use one arm to hold them and, often, the other arm to quiet them when danger lurked. With hands occupied, human females needed help. They needed fathers to stick around. One of the profound consequences of evolution, including the amusement-park-ride aspect of birth, is that it has forced humans to be interdependent and social. New mothers need help in birthing their babies—whether from an obstetrician, a midwife, a father, or an unlucky cab driver—and then they need help in bringing them up. In our modern society, that help often comes from a traditional source: fathers. But it also comes from gay or straight partners, adoptive mothers and fathers, foster families, grandparents and other family members, and loving caretakers of all sorts.

FOURTH TRIMESTER
BRAIN DEVELOPMENT

Scientists now know that the brain continues to change and grow, allowing for a lifelong ability to reorganize neural pathways based on new experiences. That ability is called neuroplasticity.[5] But while recent discoveries suggest that new neurons are produced throughout life, it doesn't happen nearly as rapidly as it does during the nine months spent in the womb. Some 100 billion neurons form during pregnancy. At birth, all those neurons are as yet incapable of communicating with each other.

But nature has made sure that the neural circuits responsible for basic body functions are up and running at birth. Infants arrive with the most basic and primitive operating equipment, under the control of the lower parts of the brain. During gestation, the basic architecture of the brain is laid down, beginning development soon after conception. That prenatal architecture eventually includes the brain stem, or lower part of the brain, regulating the central nervous system and cardiac and respiratory functions; the thalamus, two bulb-shaped masses above the brain stem that process and relay sensory information; and the cerebellum, which coordinates motor movement. Those parts direct the infant to kick, grasp, cry, sleep, root, suck, swallow, keep a heartbeat going, and manage a circulatory system. It's all primitive or immature, and the higher centers, those in charge of emotions, intelligence, planning, and motor responses, are still waiting to be formed, influenced by love, conversation, comforting touch, faces, movement, sound—in short, the world he was born into.

The work begins almost immediately. Each newborn is busy developing neural connections by laying down a network of dendrites, branched projections that receive signals of communication and pass them on with the aid of neurochemicals. The connections formed are called synapses. During the first three years of human life, there is an unprecedented pattern of rapid synapse formation. In fact, babies develop so many synapses there simply isn't room for them all, and those that aren't used go by the wayside. The ones that remain get more efficient at providing the information we need.

This is how it works. Neurons are cells specializing in sending and receiving signals. A neuron in the eye gets its signal from light; in the ear, from sound vibrations; in the nose and tongue, from molecules that bind to them; and on the skin, signals come from touch. A message travels, via electrical signal, from neuron to neuron to the part of the brain specializing in, say, seeing, tasting, or moving. Then the output side kicks in, sending an outgoing signal to the retina, or the tongue, or a muscle, complete with instructions on how to move, extend, or contract. So even as the brain is constructing a branchlike communication network, it is also beginning to pare down the number of neurons in the brain in order to ease overload, making experience key to wiring an infant's brain.

During that time, an infant's brain experiences sporadic bursts of activity that are known as exuberant periods. At the peak of one of these periods, the brain is creating 2 million new synapses every second, researchers estimate. These bursts of development happen at various times in different areas of the brain during the first months of life and continue, though at a slower pace, through adolescence.[6] During infancy, the new connections allow for color vision, the ability to grasp, and a strong attachment to parents. Each baby is sculpting a brain that is becoming truly human and uniquely his own.

Neuroscience has become adept at studying the tiny but interconnected cells of the brain using brain-imaging technology. Going well beyond earlier scientific tools—such as observation, autopsies, x-rays, and EEGs—CT scans, functional MRIs, and PET scans create three-dimensional images of the brain and allow scientists to analyze its chemical composition, its electrical transmissions, and the blood flow through the brain. Through the use of such technology, we now know that when babies are born, they come equipped with more neurons than they'll ever need, and some, but not many, synapses.

The neurons are the raw material of the brain, and heredity determines their number.[7] (Only recently has research begun to show that important areas of the forebrain continue to produce new neurons into adulthood.)[8] But the infant brain is in a remarkably unfinished state, with its billions of neurons that are unable to communicate with each other. Those connections only begin to be formed as the baby experiences the world and the love of parents and caretakers. Nature and nurture go hand in hand as each sensory interaction adds to the wiring.[9] The number of synapses skyrockets during the first three months and beyond, for as long as three years. At birth, an infant has about twenty-five hundred synapses per neuron. By three she has about fifteen thousand synapses per neuron, or some 1,000 trillion synapses—twice the number of an adult brain.[10]

It's too many, and the brain knows it, as it kick-starts a use-it-or-lose-it mechanism, a lifelong process that begins during the fourth trimester even as new connections are being made. Synapses are refined and pruned to eliminate those brain connections that are not used, and to favor those that get used frequently.[11] Coo, cuddle, and comfort a baby, and the synapses responding to loving behavior will endure. Scream, neglect, or strike a baby—events that are read by the brain as toxic stress—and the synapses responding to cruelty and violence will take hold. The brain pathways that are repeatedly used, even as early as the fourth trimester, are protected.

Caregivers' every interaction serves to support the scaffolding for infants' developing brains, part of the crucial postfetal development period that acts as a transition in getting them ready for the world. The earliest games of peekaboo form neural connections for vision as faces come close to infant faces and then disappear. The first hushed baby-talk messages begin to wire young brains for the sounds of language, specifically their own native language. Each new neural structure allows for newer layers of increasingly complex structures. Parental games, lullabies, verbal patter, and comforting touches all cause the newborn's brain to vigorously form the connections that in turn increase the number of complex links needed for passing electrochemical messages from brain neighborhood to brain neighborhood.[12] All of this biological activity mingles with every sound, touch, sight, taste, and smell that mothers, fathers, and caretakers provide. And since the environment is different for every infant, each newborn begins to be transformed into the irreplaceable baby parents have been waiting for.

THE CHANGE FROM STRANGE
NEONATE TO ONE-OF-A-KIND BABY

The change from the newborn that a mother first held in the hospital, or the infant that was first handed to an adoptive parent, to the child that is a unique part of the family doesn't happen in the delivery room. It begins to happen during the outside-the-uterus fourth trimester of development as worldly experiences shape the developing brain. What for nine months was largely under the purview of evolution and genetics now partners increasingly with culture and environment. Brain development becomes a product of a delicate balance between nature and nurture, genes and environment. Most scientists agree that the nature/nurture debate is over, and it's a tie, with each influencing the other. Genetic predispositions, while influencing brain growth, don't altogether dictate it. Non-genetic influences—neighborhood, parents, siblings, extended family, peers, school, and nutrition—are important in shaping who this special infant will become. Both nature and nurture are important.

When a mother cuddles an infant, she affects the formation of neural connections. When a father hums a lullaby, the infant's brain responds by retaining the cells that feel the pleasure of the sound. Touching, comforting, rocking, talking, and sing-ing to babies provide exactly what they need to stimulate their growing brains. As the baby is exposed to her unique surround-ings, a remarkable thing happens. The brain activity resulting from environmental influences causes synaptic connections—

neuron to neuron—to get stronger. The next time she's exposed to a similar influence, her brain cells respond more quickly and strongly. Meanwhile, those connections that aren't needed fall away. This use-it-or-lose-it model is the basis for each infant's growing individuality.

THE NEWBORN IS PREPARED

With a brain only about one-fourth ready, babies land right smack in the middle of a chaotic and messy real world. The soothing things the growing fetus had in the womb—the peace to sleep, a controlled space for exploring her own movements, the comforting external movements of her mother, the familiar muffled sounds of the household—have been abruptly snatched away. Parents and caregivers help with the transition by paying close attention to comfort. But modern science tells us that, even though the world is confusing to newborns, they've got amazing devices with which to begin sorting it all out, right from the very start.

Despite the newborn's extreme immaturity, he is well prepared. He has at his disposal an arsenal of tools for himself; and some he'll find himself using in response to signals from mother, father, or caregivers.

Survival for an infant in the fourth trimester means being constantly close to a nurturing caregiver—to the soothing touch, sound, odor, and radiated warmth provided by someone who loves and pays close attention. Newborns are naturally built and equipped by evolution to prefer their mothers, though adopted infants have proven that their allegiance changes when it must. That closeness is a vital part of the transition from womb to world. Human babies pick up on movement patterns, breathing sounds, and body heat, all of which begin to regulate hormonal releases—melatonin to help manage the sleep-wake cycle and body temperature, and cortisol to regulate blood pressure, blood sugar, and immune response.

The kinds of behaviors that come naturally to parents and caregivers around the world are just what the baby needs. Rubbing and massaging her back, stomach, or legs keeps the infant warm; stimulates respiration, digestion, and elimination; and calms her down. Mothers naturally hold their babies most often on the left side of their bodies, and babies love feeling the soothing heartbeat. Mothers, fathers, and almost all adults talk in high-pitched voices when they speak to babies, and they look their babies in the eye. They've been doing these things for millions of years—exactly the things that newborns crave.

Just as the colt is born ready to stand, a human baby is born ready to recognize another human face, the smell of her mother's milk, and the familiar sound of her voice. It's precisely because human babies are so extremely neurologically immature at birth that they are exquisitely responsive to the body cues of adults, even to the point of matching the rhythm of breathing when they rest on a person's chest. Fetal life has prepared the newborn to recognize these cues from another loving body, and the familiarity helps to ease the transition of the fourth trimester. Babies have been responding to those instinctive touches, smells, and sounds since the first human put one foot in front of the other.

"We are all preemies at birth, relative to other primates. The baby is highly sensitized to gases the mother gives off," says Dr. James McKenna, anthropologist and director of the Mother-Baby Behavioral Sleep Laboratory at the University of Notre Dame. "Every baby in the world—put them next to their mothers and they all do the same thing. They root. They breathe differently. The baby is waiting to respond to these kinds of things. They have come off a long evolutionary tree, and they know what to do."[13]

Evolution, biology, genetics, and the environment all help to fashion one special baby, far better than anything parents might have imagined. But the deep well of parental love won't be returned in kind. Not yet. Babies need that love, can't thrive without it; but at first, it's all an infant can do to handle the new work of eating, breathing, and regulating her own heartbeat and digestion. She's not yet ready to show any signs of returning the outpouring of love. It can seem like unrequited love, but the demands and frustrations of the first months do not represent a failure of parenting. It's not personal. It's simply biology. Parents have waited for a baby, and they've been handed a mysterious, not-fully-formed neonate. Patience. The baby's brain, from the moment of birth, is beginning to mature, to figure out sleeping, seeing, hearing. It's part of the dance of life—her cries, grimaces, and involuntary smiles encouraging a parental response and paving the way for a two-way attachment.[14] In time, she'll begin to respond. And one day soon, she'll smile, a reward making it all worthwhile.

WHETHER THEY KNOW IT OR NOT, PARENTS ARE PREPARED

Sometimes we describe newborns as "half-baked" or "almost finished." In many ways this is true. Fortunately, nature, evolution, and three trimesters in the womb have prepared your newborn to begin the transition to the real world during the first three months outside the uterus. In these pages, readers will come to understand the fascinating and rapidly unfolding body of research from biologists, neuroscientists, developmental scientists, evolutionary anthropologists, and physicians that both explains why this new human being is so unformed and lays out what he needs during the fourth trimester. Parents, caregivers, and health care workers will gain confidence in knowing that, just as infants are equipped—with massive help from adults—to handle the transition to life outside the womb, these adults, too, are naturally prepared to provide exactly what babies need.

Armed with knowledge of the natural workings of infants, parents will be able to sort through the advice and opinions of friends, family, physicians, and a $10-billion-baby-product-marketing industry that tries to convince people that their products will make babies happier, calmer, and most assuredly, smarter.

This is not to say the work of the fourth trimester is easy. It isn't. Babies clearly are not trouble-free. Indeed, there will be twenty-four-hour demands, and nights that feel like endless struggles. But with an understanding of infants' needs, limitations, and development during the fourth trimester, new mothers and fathers can begin their steady march down the parenting path with a maximum amount of self-assurance and a minimum amount of fear. As an understanding of one's mysterious newborn grows, so will the confidence needed to make the hundreds of daily decisions that will influence her growth and development.

Each healthy newborn is ready to begin this fascinating journey. And each loving parent and caregiver, too, has what it takes to confidently provide everything a baby needs.

CHAPTER TWO

Crying

*The Wakeup Call That Says Everything
Has Changed*

"I have never hurt him and don't believe I will, but I have had to leave the room he was in, go somewhere else and just breathe for a while, clenching and unclenching my fists," author Anne Lamott writes of her son's crying.[1]

When a baby screws up his face, squeezes his eyes shut, and throws his head back for a full-throttled wail, it's normal. Healthy newborns cry an average of one to three hours a day, though to any parent it seems like a lot more. Even a colicky baby, who cries more than three hours a day, will usually outgrow it in three to four months.

Small comfort.

The sound itself is so jarring, so unsettling, that it has qualified as torture, according to Dr. Jerome Groopman, author and chair of medicine at Harvard Medical School.[2] Quoting British social anthropologist Sheila Kitzinger, he says in his *New Yorker* article: "The sound of a crying baby . . . is just about the most disturbing, demanding, shattering noise we can hear."

But we now know that every newborn cry of life ushers in a human being who isn't quite ready to be separated from his mother's womb. It is his first and, for a while, only tool of communication to signal hunger, fear, or discomfort—needs that were effortlessly met in the three trimesters that preceded birth. His very survival during the transition that is the fourth trimester depends on this signaling cry.

THE BABY'S POINT OF VIEW

Think for a few moments about what birth is like for a newborn. If parents are overwhelmed at this time, we can only imagine the surprise of their infant. Emerging from a snug, temperature-controlled, and highly customized personal sac, she is suddenly in an alien environment. All she knows and craves—food, warmth, and security—has been left behind. In the uterus, she didn't have to ask for a thing. Now, during this phase of development that is so closely linked to her fetal life, her only way of asking is to cry. She's been a contented parasite for forty weeks, and though she's ready for life, she can handle it only with lots of help and definitely on her own demanding terms. It's up to parents and caregivers to quickly figure out what those terms are.

Her lungs fill with air for the first time, taking over respiratory function from the placenta. The amniotic fluid and mucous in the respiratory tract may not have been fully cleared by the forceful compression of the chest during birth—an even greater likelihood if the birth is cesarean—so her nose has to be cleared. Eyedrops make it hard for her immature visual system to see even the outline of her mother's face. The delivery room is filled with light, brighter than anything she's experienced before, and with sounds louder than anything she's heard before.

And yet, despite all the fussing that goes on immediately after delivery, some things are familiar to the baby. Colostrum, the first breast secretion before milk comes in, and the scent of her mother's nipples, both influenced by the food a mother eats, remind the newborn of the smells and tastes of amniotic fluid, also influenced by diet. That smell represents a sturdy bridge between fetal life and this new phase of development.

He hears mom coo, "Welcome, my boy," and the singsong, high-low pitch of the words is familiar. The sound is clearer now, without the muffling effect of amniotic fluid and layers of uterus and skin, and it's yet another bridge between "then" and "now." He understands nothing, but he's getting his first crude lesson in the yearslong effort to learn a language—that sounds make words. But for now the sounds are all strung together, and, like his mother, the baby is so exhausted from his birth adventure that he will probably fall sleep.

When he wakes, he feels something damp, but it's unlike the constant and soothing wetness of his nine-month amniotic-fluid bath. This is a wet, soggy, and perhaps chilly diaper, and he cries for help. His cries release cortisol, and his heart rate and temperature rise. He's picked up and cuddled within the warm circle of loving arms, and this feels vaguely familiar. His cries lessen. Then he is on a changing table, his clothes changed, and a dry diaper fastened around him. At the same time, he feels hunger pangs. His cries increase.

From the newborn's point of view, there's a lot to complain about. It's little wonder that, almost immediately, newborn infants add their own sounds to the mix of worldly noise around them—their cry of life. They are in an alien world and need help adjusting to it. Their cry is their first insistent request that attention must be paid, that care must be taken.

WHY NEWBORNS CRY

Babies are supposed to cry. It's the primary tool they have with which to communicate about a messy diaper, an empty stomach, and a need for reassurance or human connection. A baby's health is initially measured, in part, by a strong, lusty cry. Her cries communicate—loudly—her feelings, her needs, and her wants. Adults can't help but sit up and pay attention.

Research shows that normal, healthy infants have two cries.[3] They have a basic cry and a pain cry. The two are distinct enough to show up differently on printouts of acoustical analyses of infants' cries. The pain cry is urgent—usually high-pitched and loud. It comes on suddenly and includes long periods of breath holding. It's that pause between one loud, high-pitched *waaah* and the second outburst that puts parents on edge. They most likely are running to the infant's side as the next *waaah* comes through, signaling that the infant is still breathing. That's an instinct worth trusting. When the cry sounds like the baby is signaling pain, a physician should check to see if there's a physical cause. But an urgent cry of pain is also the cry of colic—signaling that parents might be in for a short-term, bumpy ride.

The other cry, the basic cry, is for everything else—hunger, discomfort, a need to be held. It is somewhat lower in pitch with a more gradual buildup in intensity. There are no interminable periods of breath holding, and overall, there's a less frantic sound to it.

By about six weeks, the infant has gained enough control of his vocal cords that he makes the amazing discovery that he can cry at will. Imagine the power! He is learning that this vocal tool brings someone to his side. At this point, he may not be crying for a basic need like food or a clean diaper. He may be crying because he needs attention, something he received twenty-four hours a day in the uterus.

Attention is a serious need for infants. They may need a burp, they might have gas or indigestion, or they may be getting tired. They may be too warm. They may want to move—in someone's arms, a rocking chair, a stroller, or a car seat gliding down the highway. They may simply be lonely and want the sound of a human voice or a cuddle. Or maybe it's just that fussy time of the day, and all a parent can do is try to provide comfort as the crying runs its course. That kind of attention teaches him that a caring adult is still there for him, just as his mother was always there for him during the first three trimesters, in the happy times and through the inconsolable times.

EVOLUTION HAS MADE
NEWBORNS ADORABLE FOR A REASON

There's a lot of crying and demanding coming from such a diminutive body. Researchers once held that crying was the sole biological siren that alerted and motivated mothers and caregivers to come to the rescue.[4]

Turns out, there's more going on in the initial communication. If crying were the only tie designed by evolution to connect babies' needs and mothers' responses, the human race might have died out millions of years ago. If high-pitched, incessant screaming were the only thanks mothers living in caves got for their pain and effort, they might have thrown up their hands in frustration and walked away in a huff—hang the future of the human race.

Luckily, infants have other ways of keeping caregivers hooked. Those other physical and behavioral skills, too, have been evolving over millions of years. Think "baby" and see wide eyes, round face, large head, chubby cheeks, small nose and mouth, short and thick extremities, and a plump body shape.[5] It's likely that evolution favored infants with characteristics that are universally thought of as adorable. Combine it all in one package, and we're inspired to take care of the baby's every need. In evolutionary terms, our attraction to the endearing details of this demanding being ensures the survival of the human species.

Babies of just about any species are adorable to adult humans—think kittens, puppies, and penguins. Walt Disney, Steven Spielberg, and Jim Henson understood the human nurturing reaction very well as they created some of the most beloved characters in American culture. What else could explain the appeal of creatures like Mickey Mouse with his oversized head, ET with his (her?) enormous eyes, or Elmo with his short, pudgy body?

The bottom line is that it's a good thing for the human race that babies are so adorable. Infants with waiflike eyes, plump thighs, and other classically appealing characteristics trigger activity in the reward centers of our brains. In the 1950s, the Nobel laureate Konrad Lorenz described a set of baby characteristics universally considered "cute." Those cute newborn attributes trigger a nurturing response and motivate us to respond with caretaking, Lorenz found. Our brains are wired to respond to typical baby adorableness. There is much more to our loving response than attempts to quiet those incessant wails of distress.

In 2009, a group of scientists brought technology to Lorenz's work. Using functional magnetic resonance imaging to observe brain activity, they observed the brains of a group of adults as they looked at photographs of classically cute infants. The researchers showed that the centers of the brain involved in nurturing and caretaking light up when adults look at photographs of chubby-cheeked, wide-eyed infants.[6]

It doesn't require a biological link to trigger the brain's reaction. The same response to adorable that is found in mothers and fathers is also found in all other adults and even in children. The appeal of a vulnerable infant generates a near-universal desire to help. "Can I hold her?" the older brother will ask, stretching his legs out the width of a couch as he tucks himself between pillows and promises to be very careful with her. Her very helplessness contains a survival tool that inspires mothers, fathers, big brothers and sisters, and all who gaze her way to provide care, support, and a sincere attempt to answer her needs.

There is within each of us a neurobiological explanation for why we feel the urge to take care of anything that resembles a baby—even a talking mouse, a little alien from outer space, or a fuzzy red Muppet.

A NEWBORN'S ABILITY
TO CREATE A DIALOGUE

We know that crying is a vital part of communication between mother, father, or caregiver and baby. And being adorable is an important part of the dynamic. But what else is needed to keep parents involved in the round-the-clock, sleep-robbing, often frustrating task of keeping a newborn baby alive and safe?

"After six weeks, none of us would still be here if crying were the only thing to keep us attached to our mothers," says

Dr. Heidelise Als, director of Neurobehavioral Infant and Child Studies at Children's Hospital in Boston.[7] Evolution required that infants develop other features if they were going to entice their mothers to hang in there with them. Dr. Als began looking at those evolved baby tricks by studying mother-infant interactions. She got to know mothers well enough during their pregnancies that they invited her into the delivery room. She watched, listened, and took notes as they first laid eyes on their offspring. ("You look like Uncle Louie." "You're here, and you're all mine.") She came back the next day, and the next, and the next and kept watching, all the while asking herself the same question: What impact is the baby having on the mother?

As time passed, Dr. Als found something that she didn't expect. There was a dialogue of facial expressions between mothers and newborns that immediately became a two-way street. From day one, the baby's open eyes made mother happy and inspired her words. The baby's yawn led to a winding down of the mother's words. A sneeze would elicit words of comfort. A scrunched-up face would trigger a tender laugh.[8]

Each baby, if you pay close attention, is keeping up his end of a conversation of signals, moods, and rhythms. He's helping to steer adult response, even as individual responses are teaching him to call up new conversational signals. Babies have ways of keeping the people who love and pay attention to them involved, and they'll begin the dialogue immediately with a birth mother, or with an adoptive parent or other committed caregiver, as soon as they get the chance. Those skills, refined through millions of years of evolution, prove to be enough to get the adults in their lives to put up with crying, sleeplessness, dirty diapers—and a transformation of life that new parents can't possibly have anticipated.

THEORIES ABOUT EXCESSIVE CRYING

Excessive crying happens a lot. In 10 percent to 25 percent of families, unexplained infant crying is the most common parental concern. The peak in crying time comes at about six weeks to two months, but can last until four to six months of age. Episodes of crying, nerve jangling for even minutes, can last for hours, with scarcely minutes of quiet respite.[9]

The traditional theory about excessive crying used to be that it was gas or an upset stomach. Now, unexplained and prolonged crying in the fourth trimester is seen primarily as an inability to regulate the sleep-wake cycle, or an immature ability to get to a calm state internally. An infant has normal states, ranging from deep, quiet sleep to fully awake lusty crying.[10]

Colicky or irritable babies are somewhat less organized in their initial sleep-wake cycles. While excessive crying generally peaks at about six weeks, and while, in about three months, most babies mature and possess a greater ability to calm themselves, some babies during the fourth trimester may be more sensitive to overstimulating environments. They get overwhelmed by a lot of activity in the household—a football game on the television, siblings fighting, the chaos of a routine dinner hour—and have not yet figured out how to soothe themselves and tamp down their arousal enough to fall asleep. Instead, they cry.

COLIC AND THE RULE OF THREES

Colic is defined not by physical problems but most commonly by time. A baby is considered colicky if she has unexplained crying for more than three hours a day, for at least three days a week, for three weeks running. By the time those numbers, or worse numbers, are racked up, parents are pretty stressed out.

A highly popular book, *The Happiest Baby on the Block* by Dr. Harvey Karp, suggests providing what he calls the "Five S's." Those are swaddling, side or stomach position while holding, shushing sounds, swinging, and sucking (bottle, breast, pacifier, or even a finger).[11] For some families, these work like a charm. Others need additional help.

If the numbers in the crying pattern are lower than in the colic guideline of threes, the infant may still be considered fussy in her parents' eyes. However one labels the problem, the crying will usually lessen as the infant matures in the fourth trimester and is better able to calm herself and regulate her sleep and wake cycles.

FUSSY OR COLICKY:
MOTHERS AND FATHERS NEED SUPPORT

With a truly fussy or colicky baby, parents need help. No caregiver can do it alone, and adults have to take care of themselves if they're going to be able to care for the infant. Professionals like physicians, social workers, or mental health workers can help. So can parenting groups, a mother, father, or in-law, or a friend who has survived a colicky baby. Spouses and partners can take turns giving each other a respite. All of that can amount to a schedule of relief—time to catch up on sleep, leave the house, and spend some time without infant responsibilities. Time out from parenting is a basic need, especially when a newborn cries excessively. The fourth trimester is, in the scheme of things, a short time. But it's incessantly demanding and tense.

In 2003 Dr. Linda Gilkerson founded the Fussy Baby Network at Chicago's Erikson Institute. The network has expanded to include programs in cities throughout the country, including one at Southwest Human Development's Arizona Institute for Early Childhood Development in Phoenix; one at the Children's Hospital and Research Center in Oakland, California; one operated by the University of Colorado Denver at the Children's Hospital; and another at the Boston University School of Medicine. Similar programs are being developed in the Los Angeles and Washington, D.C., areas. There are other organizations similar to the Fussy Baby Network, such as the colic clinic Dr. Barry Lester founded at Brown University in Providence, Rhode Island.

Gilkerson wanted to provide support for parents concerned about their infants' crying or temperament, a desire rooted in her experience with her own colicky son, Michael, during his fourth trimester. Dr. Gilkerson and Michael had endured an extremely difficult fourth trimester—for more than three months he cried inconsolably. There had been trips to the pediatrician, where he was declared healthy. Nothing was wrong, yet each day was unpredictable, adding to the stress. Michael would have endless crying bouts that his family came to call "Big Mac" attacks. He cried through feedings, diaper changes, and endless, futile attempts at comfort. Then a peaceful day would come, with no crying jags, followed by another day of "Big Mac" attacks. Through it all, he was a healthy baby. The diagnosis, common among babies who cry a lot, was the ill-defined "colic." After each medical trip, Gilkerson went home assured that her baby was fine. But she received no advice on how to deal with excessive crying herself: how to help her baby through it, or what to make of it. Despite the assurances of good health, he remained fussy—and there seemed to be no end in sight.

By the end of the fourth trimester, the excessive, inexplicable tears and howls were almost over. She recalls a moment of shared pleasure that was a long time coming. "He was born on April 3," Dr. Linda Gilkerson says. "I remember on July 4 [three months later], I was upstairs in the bedroom. I had my feet up like this," she says, demonstrating the classic infant-holding, knees-up posture, "and it was a moment of discovery. There was a sense of no barriers, limitless joy. I think it was just those cheeks and the sparkling eyes and the ability to sustain the engagement."[12]

She had already been hooked, in love with him since his birth, but now she felt he loved her in return. She could see it in his eyes, in his recognition of her, in his relaxed pleasure as he lay in her lap. It is a moment that all parents feel, when love moves in both directions and, for a lifetime, grows on both sides.

BABY ANNIE'S STORY:
WHAT IS WRONG WITH THIS BABY?

Annie was born to John and Courtney Bowles on September 18, 2009. She was an inconsolable bundle the moment she came home. "That first night, she cried and cried. Nothing seemed to soothe her," said Courtney. As a hospital social worker, Bowles had seen hundreds of newborns. But they seemed to sleep all the time, and she just wasn't prepared for Annie's crying. Her expectation had been that if Annie needed a diaper change, she'd cry for a few minutes, then coo with gratitude once clothed in a clean diaper. If she were hungry, she'd cry until she was fed.

Instead, she cried with a wet diaper, and continued crying with a dry diaper. She cried when she was hungry, and continued crying after she was fed. She cried when lying down, when sitting up in her infant seat, and when held this way and that.

Courtney and her husband tried swaddling, but Annie hated it, kicking through the tight wrap. Courtney talked to her, stream-of-consciousness talk that grew increasingly anxious—with an edge of fear to her voice—as Annie kept crying.

John would take her into the bathroom, the darkest room in the house, and flip on the fan, trying for a white-noise effect. They experimented with how they held her: upright with a face against her head, or in the traditional cradle position while pacing, pacing the hallway of their Chicago apartment. If something worked, they kept it up: three paces forward, quick turn, three paces back, quick turn. Cradled against an adult's pounding heart, Annie seemed to like the pacing—until one unpredictable moment when she didn't and cried some more.

"We worried that something was medically wrong," says Courtney. "Every time Annie started crying, it panicked me. It affected me to my core." After about six weeks, Courtney was crying almost as much as her baby. "I would doubt myself. I'd think, 'I don't know how to soothe my own child. I'm a failure.'" For the first five weeks of Annie's life, they were weekly regulars at her pediatrician's free walk-in clinic. Annie would be declared wide-eyed, alert, and growing normally.

Courtney's mother, who had moved in to help with the newborn, had to leave after four weeks. At six weeks, when Courtney found herself panicking the minute Annie started to cry, she decided it was time to get help. She called the Fussy Baby Network's Warmline in tears. The next day they sent an infant specialist to the Bowles home. "By the time they see us, they're at their wits' end," says Michelle Lee Murrah, infant mental health practitioner with the Fussy Baby Network.[13] They've read every parenting book they can lay their hands on, they've called their pediatricians, they may have rushed to the emergency room, they've heard the conflicting advice of their own parents, in-laws, and friends, and the baby still cries a lot.

When Murrah arrived at the Bowles's apartment, she attentively watched as Courtney and Annie did what they normally did. Courtney fed the infant and then put her on the floor. Mother and baby were down playing with the infant gym when Annie started crying. Murrah saw a yawn that Courtney missed. She wondered with Courtney what could be happening for Annie. Together, they continued to watch, and Murrah helped Courtney see Annie's sleepy signs. "She's tired," said Murrah, and suggested she put Annie down and leave her alone. Courtney had never, for an instant, let her baby go to sleep without holding her. Murrah encouraged Courtney to give her just a few minutes to see if Annie could comfort herself to sleep. The two women talked while Annie cried in her crib. Courtney said she felt guilty, inadequate, a mother who couldn't comfort her child. Within a few minutes, Annie was sleeping as the women continued to talk.

When Murrah left, Courtney practiced swaddling Annie in a looser fashion, the way she had tried with the support of the specialist—and it worked. She began to pay closer attention to Annie's yawns and other signals that she was tired, putting her down at the first signal. Courtney recalls, "I started paying attention to cues like yawning, rubbing eyes. When I thought she couldn't be tired, [Annie] was telling me she was tired. When I thought she couldn't be hungry because she just ate, she was telling me she was hungry again. It was a matter of learning how to really listen to her." Right about that time, Annie stopped crying. Not completely, of course. She just developed a normal, recognizable pattern of crying that her mother could now decode. Also, as Courtney grew less fearful and more confident, Annie could relax and feel that her mother was ably in charge.

WHAT'S THE ANSWER?

There is no magic formula. Babies are human, and all humans are different.

The first three months of a baby's life are not about training him to be an independent person. That comes later. The first months are all about helping him to shift from depending on the comfort of the womb to adjusting to the world he's been born into. What he needs to know is that when he is distressed, someone who cares about him is there—even if his problem is inexplicable. The response he gets as he makes his transition from womb to world is his first lesson in how life can be expected to respond to his woes.

Maybe an infant is telling her parents that their best-laid plans might not suit her needs. Dr. Heidelise Als, director of the Neurobehavioral Infant and Child Studies program at Children's Hospital in Boston, has seen thousands of babies and their parents. She says,

> I've seen parents, often professional, who had everything planned. They had their careers going, the house ready, the nursery ready, everything on schedule. They expected the baby to fit in.
>
> Then the baby screams, and they're befuddled and don't know what to do, because he's not doing what they want him to do. I see

that baby as a strong baby. He's asking, "Are you there for me? How much time can you make for me?"

We can be so pushed now. Women can be so focused from pregnancy on to get things scheduled. And that's not how parenting goes. That's not how growing up goes. I would prefer to support parents earlier, to tell the truth. This is a big step. This will reorganize your whole life, your whole emotional life. You'll gain a ton from it, but it's a dimension that a nonparent can't appreciate.[14]

A study of 157 infants, whose mothers recorded the duration of their crying for a full year, found that when mothers responded rapidly to crying, infants cried significantly less.[15] The sound of an infant's cry has been found to increase heart rate and blood pressure in adults, and to elicit feelings of anxiety and irritation. The common adult reaction is to run to the baby and try to relieve his distress. When a baby is described as "easy," caregivers still have increases in heart rate and blood pressure, but not as great as those in parents who describe their offspring as "difficult." According to research from the University of Michigan, those with "easy" babies were more alert and attentive to a crying infant than those with "difficult" babies. In other words, nonstop crying, excessive crying, and the crying of premature babies—which occurs at a higher and more irritating octave than that of full-term infants—can turn parents off, to the point of making them slower to respond.[16]

While that is understandable, it's important to try the opposite approach. Rather than shutting out the sound, try to provide comfort. Those attempts can be clumsy, but nevertheless they provide the kind of visual, auditory, and tactile stimulation that promotes infant development. Even the most bumbling attempts to soothe a baby, when performed as calmly and consistently as possible under jarring circumstances, have a positive effect. The infant is learning that someone important takes his distress seriously.

Newborns provide plenty of clues to how to care for them. And evolution has equipped people, whether biological parents, adoptive parents, or other adult caregivers, with the right instinctive responses: they hold their newborns close, offering soft words, kissing them tenderly, and gently stroking, warming, and feeding them. Even during interminable minutes or hours when none of it seems to be working, the comfort that is offered lays important groundwork.

PARENTS HAVE NEEDS, TOO

When an infant's crying overwhelms you, it's time to step back. I have an uncomfortable memory from my firstborn's infancy. I tucked my inconsolable daughter safely in her crib, and then trekked down two flights of stairs to our basement. I think I was crying, maybe shaking with frustration. I picked up a plastic laundry basket and hit it against a wooden support beam, and then hit it again. After a minute or two of this highly physical but harmless exercise, I was somewhat relieved, definitely spent, and more than a little ashamed. By the time Jenny was three months old, the laundry basket was ripped, tattered, and unusable.

I shouldn't have been ashamed. I didn't know it then, but I was doing exactly what experts today say is the right thing to do.

When frustration over a baby who won't stop crying gets out of control, first make sure the baby is safe, out of harm's way. Then walk away for the minutes it will take to regain calm control. Away from their infants, mothers and fathers can then do whatever makes them feel better: Clench and unclench their fists. Hit a laundry basket against a beam. Ears covered, jog in place. Call a friend, neighbor, or relative and ask for help. Do anything necessary to get the frustration out, as long as it's away from the baby. Then, relieved and refreshed, they can go back and tend to the infant's needs.

CONFIDENCE

Parents should remember: they're still the people they always were. When infants continue to cry despite all the best efforts of parents, it's easy to follow them down that rabbit hole into escalating fear and panic. But rather than take that route, it's time for parents to flex their parental muscles—not by being cold and unresponsive, but by holding on to the confidence and certainty that they're truly doing all they can. Sometimes doing all they can means simply being with the baby through moments that are particularly hard.

The infant is disorganized internally, but the adults around him don't have to be. They can take a cue from *Saturday Night Live*'s character Stuart Smalley and recall: I'm good enough, I'm smart enough, and doggone it, this baby likes me. This is true even when the baby's face is red, his stomach is tight, he's looking in all directions, and he's screaming. As mothers, fathers, and caregivers stick with it through the difficult times, they're teaching infant brains that, when in distress, help is nearby.

It helps to share calming information with a baby. *We'll get through this, sweetheart.* Remind the baby that the last time he cried for a long time, he eventually stopped and fell asleep. *Remember this morning? You cried hard then, and after a while you had a good sleep. You will again.* Mustering up a confident voice, parents can remind their infant that someone is there for him when he's happy, and remains there for him when he's distressed. In the process, those brain connections that signal comfort will be formed and strengthened; those that signal neglect will be ignored.

A confident voice sounds far different, even to an infant, than a voice shaking with uncertainty. Courtney Bowles, during those weeks when she was unable to soothe crying Annie, lost what was probably the most crucial element in her arsenal—her self-confidence. And don't think Annie didn't notice. Babies take everything in through their developing senses. When a parent's body speaks with calm conviction—the voice, the face, the movements—it must sound to an infant like reassurance.

REASSURANCE, EMPATHY, SUPPORT, AND TIME-OUTS

Reassurance is crucial for parents of colicky or fussy babies. They understandably want certainty that nothing is physically wrong with an infant who cries more than average, and this reassurance is the first step in helping parents deal with a baby who cries inexplicably and excessively. A physical checkup can rule out any health problems, but plenty of parents get that from a pediatrician or an emergency room team, only to go home with a baby who continues to cry. Parents also need reassurance that they're competent and capable of helping their infants through a trying time. Friends and family, the circle of people who know the capabilities of new parents, can be good at providing encouragement.

It's important for parents to find people who listen without judging, whether they're friends or professionals. People who work with parents of colicky babies hear the stories of parents who are at their wits' end. They hear stories of bone-wearying nights of pacing, of a midnight walk in a stroller or ride in a car seat to induce calmness. They hear confessions: *I get worked up and I'm not capable of soothing her. She feels my heart racing. She hears me crying.* They hear parents say things they're not supposed to admit: *I know I'm supposed to love him, but honestly, sometimes I feel that I don't even like him.* Parents need objective support, not harsh judgments.

"We take a lot of time to hear their stories," says Murrah of Erikson Institute's Fussy Baby Network. "We don't dismiss anything a parent says." They get SOS calls from multimillionaire parents and from housing project parents, from mothers who breast-feed and mothers who bottle-feed, from biological parents and parents who have adopted their infants. Parents of all stripes may experience the plight of sleeplessness, a lack of positive feedback from their infant, and the disappointment of limited gratification for their efforts.

The Colic Clinic at Brown University, like the Chicago Fussy Baby Network, has what it calls a Warmline to help parents. As Dr. Barry Lester notes in his book, crying is normal for an infant. It's a sign of a healthy baby who is increasing his lung capacity and generating muscle heat even as he's signaling that something is wrong. But when it goes on too long, is inexplicable, and may be endangering the parent-infant bonding relationship, it's time to ask for help.

FANTASY AND REALITY

Let's face it. The problem with any real relationship is that reality has a hard time measuring up to fantasy. No matter how much spouses love each other, are they as caring, responsive, smart, selfless, and good looking as the best either one has ever imagined? Unlikely.

So, too, the infant who arrives in the home may not quite be the one parents imagined for nine months or longer. They may have envisioned an infant who nurses calmly and gratefully, who responds to gentle touch, who gurgles sweetly as household members go about daily tasks. Instead, at times the infant fusses while feeding or turns away from a gentle touch. It's hard not to take it personally as parental confidence sags. Parents of babies who fuss and cry a lot may see other mothers strolling in the park or at the mall, and it looks to them like everyone else has calm and happy infants. They know they would never venture out in public with an infant who wrinkles up and screams as their fumbling attempts to calm him fall flat.

Babies who cry a lot and who are unresponsive to attempts at soothing need parents and caregivers to hang in there just as much as do "easy" babies. Maybe more. They're learning that they have some power in the world and will get a response, that they can make things happen, that someone cares. Eventually, the optimism that comes from having their needs met will help them calm down enough to smile, to be curious, and to begin to learn.

The calm-shattering wails of a hard-to-console baby must not become a barrier to showing love. The goal of steady and sturdy brain development is reached by making infants feel safe and loved. When parents show newborns that they are there when there's trouble—known trouble like a soiled diaper or hunger, or inexplicable trouble—infants build important neurological connections that will allow them, someday soon, to expect love, comfort, and safety when they feel afraid. As infants, they're not manipulating us. They don't yet know how.

From an infant's point of view, there is an array of things that might be amiss: She's hungry, wet, or tired. She needs to burp, or move, or be more tightly wrapped or maybe less tightly wrapped. She could be hot or cold. She might be lonely and want some company, or she may have had too much light, noise, or adult company. Maybe it's just that time of day. An intimate one-on-one loving connection with the infant during the fourth trimester, almost as close as the enforced bond during pregnancy, is what's needed for each newborn. She's helpless and she needs her mother, her father, or her consistent caregiver.

CHAPTER THREE

Sleeping

Irregular and Sporadic Sleep Is Normal in the Fourth Trimester

One afternoon, when Abigail Lee was about six weeks old, she slept for four hours. It was heaven for her mother, Molly Lee. But during the baby's fourth trimester, that one long nap was a fluke. "Usually, she sleeps for two and a half hours," says her mother. "It's stressful. Generally, when she's sleeping, I try to get a nap. But sometimes I can't sleep. Or when she's sleeping, I want to be human: answer email, clean the house. You know, try to reclaim myself a little bit."

A newborn may not be sleeping as much as his parents hoped he would, but he's sleeping exactly the way he's supposed to sleep in his first three months—irregularly, sporadically, in long and short episodes, and whenever he wants. That's what he was accustomed to doing so very recently in the uterus. Now, as he makes the transition to the world during the fourth trimester, chemicals released through proximity to mother, father, or caregiver are beginning to help the infant regulate his sleep. When, where, and how long a newborn sleeps are probably the most troubling and frustrating aspects of his fourth trimester.

Sleeping through the night is a milestone for babies—and a tremendous relief for parents. But it didn't happen in the womb, and it doesn't happen quickly during this time of transition. It takes months for an infant to sort out day from night.

With so many parents reporting that their babies have sleep problems, it's little wonder that everyone has a so-called solution. But conflicting advice from pediatricians, books, magazines, other mothers, and friends may cause mothers and fathers to see problems where none truly exist. Sleep researchers have considered the social pressure on parents to have a "good baby" who sleeps long and well, and many have concluded that few infants have real sleep problems. "Overwhelmingly, infants don't have sleep problems to solve," says Dr. James McKenna, director of the Mother-Baby Behavioral Sleep Laboratory at the University of Notre Dame. "Parents do."[1] That is, parents have a sleep expectation problem. How much an infant sleeps during the fourth trimester, and when he sleeps, is entirely up to him. He's still making the transition from the womb, where his mother's daytime movements might have rocked him to sleep, and where her nighttime inactivity caused him to stir. He needs to eat small amounts of food often—which so recently happened automatically in the uterus. Now, hunger wakes him, and he must ask for food in the only way he knows how. And his brain hasn't yet settled into a circadian rhythm that comes anywhere near resembling the twenty-four-hour clock the rest of the world obeys. Still, he knows how much sleep he needs, and he'll get it, so long as no one gets in his way.

HOW MUCH SLEEP IS ENOUGH?

It's reassuring to know that a newborn will sleep just the right amount, based on her body and individual makeup. The rule of

TABLE I

Average Sleep Duration

(hours)

Age	Total Sleep	Night Sleep	Day Sleep
1 month	14–15	8	6–7
3 months	14–15	10	4–5

SOURCE: Ivo Iglowstein, Oskar G. Jenni, Luciano Molinari, and Remo H. Largo, "Sleep Duration from Infancy to Adolescence: Reference Values and Generational Trends," *Pediatrics* 111, no. 2 (February 1, 2003): 302–307.

thumb, referred to in countless books and advocated by many pediatricians, is that newborns sleep an average of sixteen hours each day.[2] But this is the average, and there are plenty of outliers. Some parents share horror stories of how little their infants slept, especially at night, while others chirp about what a good baby they had because she slept for hours on end each night. Despite averages and anecdotes, infants during the fourth trimester have a wide range of sleep habits.

Still, there are studied averages. One of the best studies was a long-term survey of 493 Swiss children tracked from birth.[3] The results for babies at ages one month and three months are listed in table 1. But don't read too much into them. A baby could get more or less and still be healthy.

In this study, there wasn't much difference between the average amount of sleep at one month and the amount of sleep at three months, though by three months' time the infants were showing hints of sorting out day and night by sleeping two fewer hours during the day, two additional hours at night. The chart shows averages, but there was wide variation in the babies studied. During the fourth trimester, some infants in the study slept as few as nine hours in a twenty-four-hour period, while others slept as many as nineteen hours.

Since no one can tell parents how much sleep is enough for an individual baby, it's up to them to read their baby's signals. Even very young infants have ways of letting their caregivers know they're sleepy. Some of the classic clues they offer are yawning or attempting to rub their eyes or ears. They may look away from things that would normally catch their interest. They may flutter their eyelids. They're saying that it's time to go to bed.

During pregnancy, most parents no doubt keep their fingers crossed that they'll deliver one of those kids who sleep nineteen hours, even as they worry that it would be just their luck to get one who sleeps only nine hours in a day. But once she's on the scene, it's time to figure out how to deal with her unique sleep habits.

UNDERSTANDING THE SLEEP
ARCHITECTURE OF A NEWBORN

An infant's sleep looks nothing like an adult's, as seen through the squiggly lines of electroencephalograph (EEG) readings. Instead, an infant's sleep comes in spurts, some as short as thirty minutes, others lasting three or more hours. From the beginning, infants sleep as easily during the day as they do at night. After all, it's what they've been doing for nine months, and it's what they continue to need during the fourth trimester of their development.

As the newborn's body adjusts to the rhythms of the world, he will move from eight hours of daytime sleep and eight hours of nighttime sleep (those hours, of course, interrupted by feeding and wailing) during his first months to eleven to twelve hours of nighttime sleep and only two to three hours of daytime sleep. A recent study found that the appearance of some semblance of an adultlike pattern of circadian rhythm, as measured by the hormone cortisol, begins to emerge at about eight weeks.[4] But it isn't until about the six-month mark that the miracle of long stretches of uninterrupted sleep after dark begins to happen. Even that doesn't mean that sleep at night will be uninterrupted. At about a half a year, most babies begin to sleep in approximately six-hour stretches, will wake for a quick meal, and then can sleep another six hours. By one year, most babies are getting the majority of their sleep at night in one long stretch, along with one or two daytime naps.

TWO PHASES OF NEWBORN SLEEP

During roughly the first two months of the fourth trimester, a newborn's sleep is divided into two categories: active sleep and quiet sleep.[5]

1. Active sleep—For the first twenty-five minutes of sleep, an infant is in the active sleep phase. The activity is apparent in her face. She has a lot of eye movements, smiles, frowns, irregular breathing, and muscle movements. She's much more likely to awaken during this first stage of sleep, so it's best not to disturb her then.

2. Quiet sleep—An infant then moves from active sleep to quiet sleep. During this phase, she breathes rhythmically, makes sucking motions, and has very few muscle movements. This phase of sleep too lasts about twenty-five minutes.

THE FIRST MONTH

In the first few weeks of life, newborn sleep is divided about evenly between active sleep and quiet sleep, making up one complete cycle of infants' sleep architecture. And each time newborns fall asleep, they go through one or two of those cycles, giving them a sleeping time of one to two hours, though occasionally they'll sleep longer than two hours or less than an hour.[6]

A third phase of sleep, called indeterminate sleep, probably makes a brief appearance during the sleep cycle of a newborn. But it cannot be defined by today's sleep measuring technology until an infant reaches about two months of age.

Babies' sleep cycles are pretty unorganized and inefficient during the first month or so, and infants are awakened easily, especially during the first, or active sleep, phase. So while there are no guarantees, transferring a sleeping infant from arms to a crib is likely to be more successful when he's in quiet sleep. That'll be about twenty-five minutes after he falls asleep, and an attentive parent or caregiver can tell by studying him. Wait until the eyelids stop fluttering and breathing becomes more regular. He may sleep just another twenty-five minutes or so as he completes the quiet sleep cycle. But there are those lucky times, too, when he just might enter another fifty-to-sixty-minute cycle of first active sleep, then quiet sleep.

THE SECOND MONTH

At around two months of age, the circadian rhythm begins to emerge. That's the day-and-night rhythm of human life, the rhythm that signals us to get up in the morning and, hours later, to finally give it up for another day. Hormones fuel this natural rhythm: cortisol gets us moving in the morning, and melatonin makes us feel sleepy at night. At around two months, an infant's hormonal system begins to operate and her circadian rhythm will start to emerge. Now, that third phase of sleep, indeterminate sleep, can be measured on sonograms. The sucking motions and characteristic eye movements of REM sleep begin to appear later in the sleep cycle, after about thirty to forty-five minutes. What had been an immeasurable period of indeterminate sleep during the first couple of months begins to organize into the adultlike sleep patterns.

By about two months, an infant will begin to notice the environmental cues of light and dark and the different routines surrounding day and night feedings. During this month she'll begin to get slightly more of her sleep at night, slightly less sleep during the day. During the second month, the infant's brain will get a little better at organizing day and night, though this may not produce much relief for parents yet.

THE THIRD MONTH

Around three months of age, an infant's sleep cycle on an EEG starts to look a lot more like that of an older child or adult. His active sleep, equivalent to adult REM sleep, when dreams appear, is arriving toward the end of his sleep cycle, not the beginning. Since that's the time he'll wake up more easily, caregivers, starting when he's about three months old, might begin transferring him from their arms to his bed soon after he falls asleep, rather than waiting twenty-five minutes or so as they did during the first two months. Clues will continue to present themselves in his face and body. Still eyelids and regular breathing are signs that sleep is likely deep enough to risk a move.

Babies' early sleep cycles are difficult for parents to get through, but this extreme disorganization of sleep serves babies' survival needs. Babies need nourishment more than anything, and they need it with insistent regularity. That, of course, is one thing that wakes them up. But there are other things: wet diapers, a chill in the air, or too much warmth. Or it could be that they sense being alone, and after forty weeks in the uterus, they're not used to solitude. In evolutionary terms, it hasn't been long since even a brief separation from the parent meant certain death. Little wonder that infants come into this world ready to protest isolation, day or night.

DISTINGUISHING DAY FROM NIGHT

Even very young infants average slightly more sleep at night than they do during the day. Parents can help them along. Newborns pick up on the daily activities within the household when they're included in those activities. Letting a baby hear adults rattling around in the kitchen in the morning, even if it means he's asleep in a playpen in a busy room full of morning activity, will teach a baby that daylight means: get moving. Including him on the day's errands, even if he's sawing logs in a Baby Björn, is another lesson that daytime is for activity.

Environmental cues, too, can teach infants that things quiet down at night. Quiet evening feedings, with no television, in dim light, and with as little noise as possible, give them lessons in day's end. Routines, like a bedtime bathing ritual followed by a change to pajamas and some time spent being gently rocked or sung to, will begin to let them know that dark means night, and night means sleep.

When infants wake frequently, they don't have a sleep problem. "They're just sleeping like babies," says infant sleep researcher Dr. James McKenna.

LOOK FOR SIGNALS

Infants are fully capable of communicating their need to sleep. It's up to parents and caregivers to pay close attention as they learn to read those signals. It's the infant's timetable, and nobody else's, that counts during the first three months of life. A big yawn is a universal signal that someone is tired, but newborns have other common signals, too. They rub their eyes or ears. They open and close their hands. They avert their eyes, as though they're saying "no" to the stimulation of the world. These initial signs of sleepiness offer an opening to parents or caregivers to help the baby by quieting down his surroundings and gently rocking him or talking to him softly.

Problems with sleeping and excessive crying go hand in hand. Recall Courtney Bowles, who sought help from the Fussy Baby Network of the Erikson Institute in Chicago because baby Annie was seemingly inconsolable. Courtney was shocked during the first home visit from a network nurse. Mother and baby, who had just been fed, were playing on the floor when the nurse suggested that Annie was tired. "I thought she couldn't be tired. She's only been up for forty-five minutes," says Courtney. "There's no way on earth she needed another nap that soon." What the nurse saw, and Courtney overlooked, was that Annie yawned. When Courtney put Annie down, she went to sleep with little fuss. Annie had her own internal timetable, and it didn't follow a clock.

THE FIVE *S*'S

Helping a baby to sleep, both physicians and sleep researchers agree, boils down to recreating the snug, womblike environment that the newborn left so suddenly at the end of the third trimester. Science has not yet been able to precisely produce an artificial uterus. If that were possible, the problem of preterm delivery could be solved. For a full-term infant, such an exact reproduction is not what's needed. Rather, infants need one foot in the former world of the uterus, and one foot leading the way to the future.

One way to ease the transition is Dr. Harvey Karp's strategy, providing the five *S*'s: swaddling, side or stomach position while holding, shushing sounds, swinging, and sucking.[7] Let's look at just one aspect of that comfort from a newborn's perspective. Before birth, he could kick with ease, his movements contained by the soft boundaries of the womb. No sooner would he start testing the motion of a limb than the confines of his mother's body would halt the movement. After birth, he might try those same tests of movement with no uterine wall to stop him. As one leg flies up or an arm shoots out, the movement takes his body places he's never been before. He startles himself awake. Here's where Karp's first *S* comes in. By swaddling the infant, his parents provide him with almost the comfort of the womb, the tight wrap preventing him from waking himself up with his uncontrollable movements. Legions of parents have successfully navigated through sleep issues in the fourth trimester by following Dr. Karp's guidance.

EXPECT CHANGE

Ingenious (or desperate) parents—or any others who have accompanied an infant through a sleepless night—have come up with elaborate sleep solutions that work perfectly—until they don't. A few examples show that creative juices can be unleashed by sleepless nights.

David and Sasha Kier were sure that they had figured out how to get Rocco, their one-month-old, to fall asleep before his dad and mom fell apart. David would bring a large exercise ball into the bathroom, turn on the shower, and hold Rocco while bouncing on the ball and listening to the rhythm of the running water. "It works like a charm," he declared after one week, ecstatic that he'd found the key to soothing his son to sleep. A week later, he and Sasha were despondent. Rocco was no longer interested in being bounced to sleep while listening to running water. David then started to walk Rocco around the neighborhood in his carriage until he fell asleep. It wasn't unusual to see the two of them on a midnight walk. In his own way David was soothing and waiting for sleep to overtake his newborn. When a rainstorm disrupted this activity, David moved Rocco into the car seat and drove around and around the block, but moving him from the car into the crib became a game of timing. David and Sasha were learning that there was no simple magic solution.

Infants, like anyone else, must find the process of learning, and the brand-new synapses that go along with it, exhilarating. But also like anyone else, they probably find endless repetition boring. Bouncing on an exercise ball, when new, is pretty interesting. Hour after hour of bouncing, day after day, might leave them wanting another new experience from their environment.

There are countless individual differences in the things that lull and soothe babies. Jack Doncette couldn't sleep as a newborn without swaddling. "His arms and legs just kept going and going," said his mother, Danielle. He also liked the outdoors and was lulled by the sight of swaying branches with leaves. So it wasn't unusual to see Danielle walking beneath a canopy of trees, waiting for Jack's eyelids to get heavy.

Newborns give signals, and it's up to those who love them to recognize the clues. Abigail, daughter of Molly Lee, who lives in Silver Springs, Maryland, spent a couple of days in the neonatal intensive care unit (NICU) after she was born. The baby had been projectile vomiting; happily, monitoring showed nothing seriously wrong. By the time Molly brought Abigail home from the hospital, she believed she could identify the look of fear in her newborn's face, a look that she first observed in the NICU. "One night, I was exhausted and wanted her to go to sleep after I fed her," says Lee. "I put her down, but then I looked at her face and saw that fearful look that I saw in the NICU. Tired as I was, I picked her up, held her, and she went back to sleep." Even though Abigail was in the chaotic first month of the fourth trimester, Molly was able comfort her until she relaxed enough to fall asleep. The episode likely eased Abigail through the transition of the fourth trimester. She was used to company and comfort in the uterus. She craved it again as a newborn, all the more because of her NICU experience, and Molly was able to recognize the need and accommodate it.

They're all different. Some love swaddling, others won't stand for it. And their preferences will change. My grandson, inconsolable one evening as I babysat him, finally settled into sleep when I went into the kitchen—lit only by the clock lights on the stove and microwave—held him tightly to my chest, and gently swayed back and forth. The next time I tried it, he continued to fuss. Then a friend, helping me babysit, took over. She took him into a darkened room and talked softly as she paced. He fell asleep. Not only are all infants different, but also each one will respond differently to soothing attempts almost every time they're tried.

CRYING IT OUT

Letting an infant one, two, or three months old cry and cry is a terrible idea. It means that the adults who are charged with paying round-the-clock attention are ignoring the baby's only means of communication. Infants are not physically or emotionally ready to sleep several hours through the night until about the age of four to six months. They may not be ready, during parts of the day or night, to sleep more than an hour or two. Even the kind and gentle sleep-training technique of allowing the baby to cry for a time, entering the room to pat and reassure her, then leaving her again to cry—in each instance lengthening slightly the time the baby is alone—is meant for older babies, not for newborn infants.

When a baby is awake during the fourth trimester, she needs attention, whether it's a clean diaper, a feeding, the sound of a recognizable voice, or the feel of a familiar touch. She had all her needs instantly met for a recent forty weeks, and she needs to know they'll still be met—as instantly as possible.

BABY'S FIRST BEDROOM

Should the newborn move in with mom and dad? Or should he go straight to a room of his own? The answer is often dictated more by societal expectations than by science. In Japan, the majority of newborns sleep with their parents. In the United States, many babies have a crib waiting for them in their own nursery room.

But recent recommendations by the American Academy of Pediatrics don't support the idea of a separate bedroom for newborns. Infants should sleep near, though not with, their mothers and fathers, according to the AAP. Sleeping close enough for a comforting touch during the night is ideal. And a recent study suggests why. Researchers measured heart rate variability in sixteen two-day-old infants when the babies were sleeping alone and when they were touching the skin of their mothers. The measurements were taken at one-hour intervals while the infants were still in the hospital. They had more nervous system activity, and less quiet sleep, when they were separated from their mothers. The authors suggest that the newborn may not be well equipped to cope with sleeping alone.[8]

Still, practical questions about cosleeping remain, and Dr. James McKenna, an anthropologist who is director of the Mother-Baby Behavioral Sleep Laboratory at the University of Notre Dame, has done innovative studies of mothers and babies sleeping together and apart. Bodily contact between mothers and infants, he argues, based on his research, has been evolving for thousands of years in order to keep newborns protected and fed.[9]

Dr. McKenna's passion for scientific evidence about infant sleep began with the birth of his son, Jeffrey, in 1978. He laid the infant on his own chest. "I saw that I could manipulate his breathing," he says. "His breathing would either slow down or move faster, depending on my own breathing."

That observation was a defining moment for Dr. McKenna and his then-colleagues at the Sleep Disorders Laboratory of the University of California, Irvine, School of Medicine. This personal observation set the direction for McKenna's future research. He had already been involved in the study of primates, but now he began to study the sleep of infant humans in the context of the human family.

At the Sleep Disorders Laboratory, Dr. McKenna conducted the first sleep lab studies of breast-feeding mothers and their infants.[10] He found that there were physiological and behavioral differences between mother and baby when they shared a bed compared to when they slept alone. Breast feeding and cosleeping, when done correctly and safely, go hand in hand, according to McKenna's studies.[11] A baby's proximity to an adult during sleep changed the sleep architecture of both mother and baby, and it helped infants regulate their own physiological patterns, like breathing and body temperature. Contact with adults in bed also helps to begin to regulate the release of the hormones cortisol and melatonin—the hormones that help baby begin to set her biological clock to differentiate day and night. Additionally, both mothers and babies spent less time in deep sleep, and more time in light sleep, when they slept together than they did when McKenna tested the same mother and infant pairs as they slept alone. Additional time in light sleep, he theorizes, keeps babies safe because mothers are quickly aroused by even slight movements and noises from their infants.

SLEEP AND SIDS

Although the causes of SIDS (sudden infant death syndrome) haven't all been fully defined, many researchers believe that one factor is a deficient arousal mechanism in some infants during deep sleep, which renders them incapable of recovering from the short breathing stoppages that all infants experience.[12]

When an infant is in or near her parent's bed at night, a parent's breathing sounds help her to regulate her breathing, a key part of the fourth trimester transition. Any caregiver can test this out. Put the newborn on your chest, and soon her breathing will begin to match your own, because newborns are highly sensitized to the breathing of others. They'll even change the pattern of their breathing when placed next to a breathing teddy bear, a toy designed to produce artificial sounds of inhalation and exhalation.

Infants and their parents, especially their breast-feeding mothers, communicate wordlessly all through the night if they sleep in close proximity. And a recent study showed that breast feeding reduced the risk of SIDS by 50 percent at all ages throughout infancy. The authors of that study urge that women be advised to breast-feed for six months in order to reduce the risk of SIDS.[13] Breast-feeding mothers and newborns mimic each other's movements, arousals, and even heartbeat and breathing. They are intimately alert to each other's bodies, just as they were during pregnancy. Breathing sounds, the smells of another human, radiated heat, and cues from movement and touch all act to regulate breathing and can somewhat rouse the sleeping infant. Such arousals become a defense against SIDS.

BED SHARING AND
COSLEEPING: CRUCIAL DIFFERENCES

Cosleeping is not the same as sharing a bed with the baby. The American Academy of Pediatrics advises against bed sharing, but supports sleeping in close proximity to newborns. Dr. McKenna defines cosleeping as any situation in which a baby sleeps within sensory range of the mother.[14] Sensory range simply means that the mother or father can hear, see, and smell the baby—and are within easy touching distance. The infant, too, can hear, see, and smell her parents. The infant can be close to the parents' bed, but not necessarily in it.[15] This opens the door to all kinds of possibilities: a crib next to the bed, a cosleeping bassinet that butts up against the bed but gives the infant her own safe surface, or a "safe spot" in bed with mom and dad.

Throughout the twentieth century, infants were pushed farther away from their parents at night. Society was evolving to emphasize autonomy and independence, and people wrongly thought that independence could be fostered from birth by putting newborns into cribs in their own rooms.[16] But the move out of the parental bedroom failed to take into account what infants truly need—constant and immediate reassurance that the comfort, nourishment, and warmth they were used to in the womb remain nearby.

The newborn's most fundamental body makeup—heart rate, body temperature, breathing, sleep, and arousal—are highly influenced by proximity to caregivers. Stroking and massaging a human infant is akin to licking among other mammals—minus, of course, the rough-textured mammalian tongue. If an infant is within arm's reach during the night, a tender touch may be all he needs to drift back to sleep, while it barely disturbs the parents' own sleep. Touch warms the baby even as it aids breathing, digestion, and elimination. As the infant sleeps nearby—preferably touching distance away—those comforting and health-promoting rubs and pats can happen all through the night.

Sharing the same bed with parents might make sense for breast-feeding mothers. That was the norm for millions of years, until the twentieth century and the advent of infant formula, along with cultural pressures to attempt to create independent children by putting them in their own rooms immediately. (In reality, quickly anticipating or responding to an infant's needs for food, comfort, and attention fosters independence. Forcing them to wait for what they really need makes them become even more demanding. Imagine being hungry and being denied food; being wet and being denied dry clothes; or being afraid and being denied reassurance. Surely, it would make us all scream ever louder for what we need.)

A lot of parents ignore the recommendation to avoid sleeping with their babies. About half of all parents say they bring their babies into the family bed for all or part of the night.[17] They do it despite the American Academy of Pediatrics' recommendation against the practice because, during the ninety or so nights of the fourth trimester, it just makes sense now and then.[18] The newest AAP guidelines, published in 2011, continue to advise against sleeping in the same bed with an infant because, according to the AAP press release, "babies who sleep in the same bed as their parents are at risk of SIDS, suffocation or strangulation. Parents can roll onto their babies during sleep or babies can get strangled in the sheets or blankets."[19] The advice to *never* bring an infant into the family bed is at odds with many mothers' instincts to be close to their babies. But the conflict with the pediatricians' parenting guideline sets those women up to feel guilty about sharing their bed. Worse, in doing it spontaneously and guiltily, they may end up doing it incorrectly, without regard to safe bed-sharing techniques.

To be clear, cosleeping—sleeping in a separate bed but close enough that parents and babies are aware of the other's sounds, smells, and movements—is safe, healthy, and beneficial to babies and their parents. Bed sharing is in some circumstances safe, dangerous in others.

- Infants don't belong in a parental bed if one of the parents is intoxicated—with either drugs or alcohol—or if either parent smokes.

- They shouldn't share a bed with a parent who is overly exhausted and who may not be alert to the baby's sounds and movements.

- A mother who smoked during pregnancy should not sleep in the same bed as her infant, since the infant may have been born with a decreased ability to arouse himself during the normal breathing stoppages that occur. Exposure to secondhand smoke, too, may compromise the infant's ability to arouse himself.

- Other toddlers, children, or pets should never be in the same bed with an infant.

- Breast-feeding mothers and babies have increased sensitivity to each other's movements, touch, breathing, and temperature, which protects babies from overlay, or having a parent's body weight inadvertently block the infant's breathing. Bottle-fed babies and their mothers don't experience that greater sensitivity, so these babies are safer in their own spaces, near their parents' beds.

SAFE BED SHARING
FOR BREAST-FED BABIES

Where baby sleeps is an intimate family decision. Here are ways to ensure a breast-fed infant's safety when parents want the baby in their bed.[20]

- Just as they would in their own cribs, babies in their parents' beds should sleep on their backs, on a firm mattress, and without pillows, blankets, or stuffed toys near their faces. Keep in mind that almost all adult mattresses, even those called "firm," are softer than crib mattresses.

· Ideally, the bed should be pulled away from the wall so that the infant cannot tumble into the area between wall and bed. Modern adult beds are not designed for safe infant sleeping; be sure the headboard and footboard are tight against the mattress so the infant can't get wedged in small spaces. Better yet, put the mattress or a futon on the floor in the middle of the room.

· Don't use a heavy or feather-stuffed comforter. Light blankets are best, pulled up only to his chest. Warm, snuggly pajamas can eliminate the need for any kind of blanket.

· Couches, recliners, waterbeds, and stuffed chairs are dangerous because there are too many spaces in them where infants can become wedged or trapped. Some women, warned against bed sharing and unaware of safe bed-sharing procedures, still want to sleep with their infants, and so fall asleep on the couch with the baby, or in a recliner—both of which are far more dangerous than safe bed-sharing in the family bed.

· When breast-feeding a baby in bed, make sure she sleeps on her back when feeding is over.

IT GETS EASIER

In addition to worrying that their newborn isn't getting proper sleep, parents are in the throes of their own sleep deprivation. They're feeling cranky even as they're still opening congratulatory cards showing mother, father, and baby in blissful, rested contentment.

Despite their own exhaustion, they remain obsessed with the wonder of this new family member, preoccupied with his comfort and well-being. When they could be sleeping, they can't resist tiptoeing to him for just one more peek. About all they can do is hang on to their hats—and their sanity—as they try to help their newborn get enough sleep while getting enough themselves.

It won't happen overnight. In the most difficult moments, it may help to remember that an infant's needs are real and immediate, and that, in time, life will get easier.

CHAPTER FOUR

Feeding

Breast Milk and Formula

I have two daughters, and each has three children. Jenny breast-fed her babies for most of their first year, and loved it. Rachel tried breast feeding with each baby for various lengths of time—the first for nine months, the second for a week, the third for three months—and then switched to formula. She never enjoyed breast feeding.

Already, I know there are people who will say of my formula-feeding daughter: "But she didn't try hard enough," or "It's not about her pleasure," or worst of all, "She has chosen to shortchange her own children."

Feelings run high when it comes to breast feeding, and judgment can be harsh. When Kathryn Blundell wrote "I Formula Fed. So What?" in the July 23, 2010, issue of *Mother and Baby*, readers called her a "dumb tart" and told her she wasn't fit to be a parent. In her article, she wrote of a stranger in a park who approached her as she was feeding her son from a bottle. The stranger asked an impertinent, none-of-your-business question: Are you breast-feeding? (The bottle could have contained expressed milk.) When the answer was no, the intruder said, "You know, your baby will get sick if you give him that poison."

In this chapter, I want to walk a balanced line between acknowledging the superior benefits of breast feeding and breast milk (two separate concepts) while also allowing that formula is an acceptable alternative. Food, for nine months passively received by the infant, now requires effort, and it's clear from both evolution and biology that breast feeding is the most seamless and natural transition from the uterus through the fourth trimester. But no one way of doing *anything*, including feeding, is right for all mothers and families. Real-life decisions are not based on science alone, and the world is populated with billions of people who were formula-fed and lived to tell the tale. Women make the decision to breast-feed based on culture, circumstance, and their own preference—all highly personal considerations, and all of which count. A clear understanding that breast feeding provides the most natural extension of pregnancy is the starting point as each woman makes her own decision.

My six grandchildren are healthy, happy, well adjusted, and perfectly wonderful. If I had to isolate their collective multitude of charming, endearing qualities and assign credit for some to an early history of breast feeding while connecting other traits to formula feeding, I couldn't do it. Nor could anyone else.

Breast is best. But formula or breast milk in a bottle held by an adult who provides smiles, touch, gentle words, lullabies, and lots of love and attention is an excellent alternative.

SOME BASIC SCIENCE

An observed *link* between two things doesn't prove that one caused the other. Advocates of breast feeding say that mother's milk is responsible for a host of benefits for the infant, including higher IQ and a reduced risk of obesity, diabetes, high cholesterol, leukemia, and allergies.

But science has become skeptical of those black-and-white, good-or-evil comparisons of breast milk and formula. Close examination of the existing research shows inconsistent results, and benefits that are minimal at best, though recent studies present convincing evidence that breast feeding can help protect infants from SIDS.[1] Some studies show a relationship to, say, a reduced risk of allergies among breast-fed babies, while others show none.[2]

The reason for the lack of simple clarity is that the studies come largely from the field of science called epidemiology, or observational studies. Epidemiologic studies show patterns among groups, usually based on information gleaned by asking people what they have done in the past—whether they breast-fed or formula-fed—and then comparing the prevalence of disease between the groups. Or researchers might watch two groups of infants over a period of time—one group fed breast milk, the other fed formula. They would then compare disease rates between the two groups. If, say, the formula-fed infants have a higher rate of obesity, then the study has shown an association between formula and obesity.

The problem comes with the countless variables that might have entered the picture between the time of infant feeding and the time the child is deemed overweight. In addition, mothers who breast-feed have, in general, different characteristics than mothers who formula-feed. Breast-feeding moms are more often older and better educated. A college-degreed mother is twice as likely to breast-feed. In other words, the studies are confounded by demographics. A formula-fed child born into poverty has a higher risk of obesity, diabetes, and host of other problems that can be more clearly linked to poverty than to formula. And children, breast or bottle fed, born into wealthy households have advantages on many fronts, including health care and education.

One 2001 study on obesity, for example, looked at weight and infant-feeding information for about twenty-six hundred American children ages three to five.[3] Researchers wanted to know what effect early breast feeding had on future weight. After they controlled for factors like the mothers' educational level and health, they reported that they "failed to find an association between breast or formula feeding and body composition in early childhood." What they did find, however, was an association between the mother's body mass index and her baby's weight. If mom was overweight, there was a greater chance her child would be, too.

Still, there are advantages for infants who are fed breast milk, even if the evidence is not life-and-death dramatic. And there are further benefits from the intimate act of breast feeding that are at least as important as the nutrients in the milk itself.

COLOSTRUM

The benefit of breast feeding starts with the first milk to come in, called colostrum. Mammary glands begin producing it late in pregnancy and throughout the first few days after giving birth. Colostrum is high in carbohydrates and protein, as well as antibodies to protect infants from infection. It's highly concentrated, and a low volume delivers a big bang of nutrients. It carries smells similar to those in amniotic fluid, naturally easing the newborn through the transition to life.

Colostrum sets off a chain of healthy effects in a newborn's body. As a mild laxative, it encourages baby's first stool. That, in turn, clears excess bilirubin, which are dead red blood cells present at birth. The reduction in bilirubin helps prevent jaundice, or yellowing of the skin. Colostrum also contains antibodies called secretory immunoglobulin. These antibodies line infants' guts, adding to a host of antibodies already there at birth. The additional dose further protects against infection. In fact, secretory immunoglobulin has been found to especially protect premature babies. Preemies fed formula tend to vomit more than those who had that early dose of colostrum.

Formula is developed to mimic breast milk as closely as possible but cannot replicate colostrum. The early benefits from colostrum are significant, so breast feeding for even a short time is beneficial.

HEALTH BENEFITS OF BREAST MILK

The strongest evidence of further health benefits from breast milk comes from a series of studies done in 2001.[4] Dr. Michael Kramer of McGill University in Montreal came up with a unique study design. He followed seventeen thousand infants in Belarus throughout their childhoods. Dr. Kramer recruited mothers, all of whom began breast-feeding their infants at birth. But half the mothers were given education and support that encouraged them to breast-feed longer and exclusively for several months. He found that gastrointestinal infections—vomiting and diarrhea—were reduced by 40 percent in the infants who breast-fed longer.

A follow-up study published in 2008 found that the Belarus children who were breast-fed longer scored about six points higher on IQ tests and, at the age of about six and a half, were rated more highly in reading and writing by their teachers.[5] However, Dr. Kramer found no significant difference in weight, ear infections, allergies, or respiratory infections between the babies who were exclusively breast-fed and those who were fed formula. But that may be because all the babies in his study were breast-fed initially for at least a short time.

SIBLING DIFFERENCES

Are there differences between siblings when one was nursed on breast milk and another drank formula from a bottle? Maybe the way to tease out differences between breast-fed and formula-fed infants is to study such siblings. That's what economists Eirik Evenhouse and Siobhan Reilly of Mills College in Oakland, California, did.[6] Their starting point was an examination of earlier observational studies suggesting that formula-fed infants had greater rates of ear, respiratory, and gastrointestinal infections, and that they were more likely to have allergies or to be hospitalized. Some of these earlier observational studies also found that, as older children, those not breast-fed were more likely to get cancer, be obese, or develop diabetes. And a number of these observational studies claimed that formula feeding could lay the groundwork for late-life high blood pressure and heart disease.

Frightening scenarios, all. But then Evenhouse and Reilly examined the existing research through a different lens. Using data from the federally sponsored National Longitudinal Study of Adolescent Health, they compared pairs of siblings, one of whom had been breast-fed, the other formula-fed. They found no significant differences in all these areas of health and well-being, from infancy through the teen years.

They did find a slight bump in IQ among the siblings who had been breast-fed as infants. That bump was also seen in an earlier analysis of twenty separate studies on breast feeding and IQ, which found that breast-fed babies end up with a three-point IQ advantage—up to an additional five points for premature babies.

No one knows if it's the milk itself that accounts for the difference in future IQ. It could be components, such as fatty acids, in mother's milk. Or it could be simply that, overall, breast-feeding mothers interact more with their babies than formula-feeding mothers.

Scientists have recently found that breast feeding did not influence the number of infections in infants, but rather their severity.[7] It could be that breast milk does not prevent infection but instead helps infants cope better with infection.

In 2007, a group of experts prepared a report for the U.S. Department of Health and Human Services in which they examined four hundred studies undertaken in developed countries relating to the health effects of breast milk.[8] The report concluded that breast feeding is *associated* with a reduced risk of ear infections, stomach upset, asthma, childhood leukemia, and SIDS. It found no association with future IQ, and an unclear association with heart disease and overall mortality. The key word is *associated*, which means that the studies have not proven that breast feeding is directly responsible for better health. The authors concluded that, while there's a link between breast feeding and better health, the studies reviewed were observational, and so "one should not infer causality." It comes down to a basic problem: the presence of too many variables over too long a time makes it impossible to say that it's breast milk itself that leads to better health.

So it seems that the hardest scientific evidence says that breast feeding reduces incidents and severity of vomiting and diarrhea. It might add a few IQ points. Proof that it reduces future problems like heart disease, cancer, diabetes, and obesity is weak. The benefits of breast milk are real, but they are small.

Dr. Adriano Cattaneo, a pediatric epidemiologist who is also a supporter of breast feeding, wrote in the *Journal of Pediatrics and Child Health:* "We do not need to use weak and shaky arguments to convince mammals to breastfeed. What we need is effective care to let them breastfeed as much and as long as they wish."[9] Wise words. Let's not overstate the benefits of breast milk. Let's also not use scare tactics about the risks of formula. And as a society, let's support whatever choice a mother makes.

BREAST FEEDING BENEFITS

Babies are designed to breast-feed all day and through the night. It's a completely natural process that keeps babies close to their mothers while they complete the fourth trimester of development. Whether one credits this design to Mother Nature, biology, evolution, or God, it is incontestable. "It's as true as birth itself," says Dr. James McKenna, director of the Mother-Baby Behavioral Sleep Laboratory at the University of Notre Dame. "Babies are born needing a physical relationship."[10] The baby absorbs and responds to the heat of the mother, to her heart rate, her blood-pressure rate, and her levels of the hormones cortisol and oxytocin. It is birth mothers and babies who have been studied, but infants will no doubt respond to proximity to other adults who hold them closely.

During the fourth trimester, the physical relationship fostered by holding an infant to the bare skin of the breast translates over the first weeks and months to a bonding relationship for both mother and baby. The magnificent design and flow of pregnancy, birth, and breast feeding is the starting point in making a decision about how to feed an infant. It doesn't have to be the end point, but parents should understand that breast feeding is the natural biological transition from womb to world.

Economics can step in and present obstacles to nursing, such as a need for the mother to return to work. Culture can present obstacles like a lack of support for breast feeding. Medical problems can present obstacles such as a mother's need to take a pharmaceutical, making it impossible to nurse. Adoptive parents cannot naturally breast-feed. For any number of personal reasons, a woman can reasonably make a decision to formula feed, but it's important for her to know that nature's starting point at birth is to continue the process of infant development aided by breast feeding. With that knowledge, a formula-feeding parent can come close to mimicking with a bottle the closeness and intimacy of breast feeding.

NEWBORNS WANT
THEIR MOTHERS' BREASTS

Some things are undeniable, and you just can't quarrel with the breast crawl, first described in 1987 at the Karolinska Institute in Sweden. Since then, the images of newborns, minutes old, creeping up their mothers' chests have been captured in heart-warming, awe-inspiring videos.[11] The pattern is the same for all infants in the rare circumstance where they have been placed immediately on their mothers' abdomens—before all the amniotic fluid is cleaned off. First, the newborns lie still. Within fifteen minutes, they begin rooting and sucking. In about a half an hour, many try bringing their hands toward their mouths. In less than an hour after their birth, they've struck gold, finding the nipple and sucking.

Few newborns in America have the opportunity to do the crawl. After all, it's hardly part of the delivery room experience to delay cleaning and weighing for the time that the breast crawl takes. But at least one hundred newborns have been observed under research conditions around the world, and virtually all of them completed the crawl from belly or chest to nipple.

How do they know where to go? It's probably the smell of mom's body, familiar from the uterus and stronger around the area of her nipples. The nipple is rich in glands that most likely secrete smells attractive to the infant. The studied newborns were only superficially cleaned, and amniotic fluid was left on their hands. The fluid smells much like the odor secreted by mothers' mammary glands, and the reminder may spur infants to get closer to the breast. In addition, being on the mother's soft body probably provides the comfort to allow the baby to be still, begin to notice the odor, and start to try some of the kicks and other movements practiced in the womb.

Visual cues can play a role. Science has shown that newborns are attracted to contrast and to their mothers' faces. Her face is up there, above the breast, and the breast itself has the natural contrast of lighter breast and darker nipple. While the contrast is stronger in lighter-skinned women, all women's breasts have a nipple that is somewhat darker in color than skin. In addition, the infant is no doubt hearing her heartbeat and the soft sound of her voice, both sounds urging him upward.

The newborn's drive to get to the nipple indicates a strong human urge for breast feeding that goes beyond a need for the actual nutritional content of the milk.

ONE OF LIFE'S SIMPLE PLEASURES

Few experiences in life can be as rewarding as nursing an infant, provided both mother and baby enjoy the process. Some mothers, in fact, are maybe a bit embarrassed by just how *gooood* it feels. More sensual than sexual, the good feeling is triggered by hormones whose job it is to make the experience pleasant enough to encourage women to stick with it.

Prolactin is the hormone that stimulates the body to produce milk. It also helps people relax. During breast feeding, another hormone, oxytocin, is released in the mother's body, causing milk to be released from the ducts. Oxytocin plays a part in the pleasure contractions experienced during orgasm. Little wonder the experience, for many women, feels darn good. The hormone has been shown to reduce anxiety and increase feelings of calmness and security.

Mothers who breast-feed tend to touch their infants more during feedings and spend more time looking into the babies' eyes. Mothers who bottle-feed are just as capable of that kind of tactile nurturing, but research shows it's more common among breast-feeding mothers. Frankly, though, nursing is in some ways just a whole lot easier. There are no bottles to wash, no formula to mix, no nipples to sterilize, and nothing to pay for—with the significant exception of a mother's exclusive time. Supportive partners can assist nighttime feedings. Fathers can get up when their babies cry and bring them to their mothers to nurse.

WHEN BREAST FEEDING DOESN'T WORK

It's not *failure* if breast feeding doesn't work. Molly Lee breast-fed her daughter, Abigail, for eleven weeks, but ran into trouble at about three weeks. Abigail would come on and off her breast, crying and clawing. Molly gave up dairy and soy, and Abigail did better. But Molly didn't. Already a vegetarian, she grew so anxious at monitoring her diet intensely that she lost interest in food. Eating poorly set up a cycle of low energy, lack of sleep, and anxiety that eventually sent her, dog-tired and skinny, to the emergency room. When a doctor prescribed antianxiety medication, she was forced to abruptly stop breast feeding. "It killed me, but Abigail adjusted amazingly well to a specialized, dairy-free, soy-free formula. Overall, outside of the difficulty, I loved breast feeding, and Abigail was very good at it."

Discomfort, whether from breast engorgement, cracked or infected nipples, or anxiety like what Molly Lee felt, is a common reason that women discontinue breast feeding. But perhaps the most common reason is that women go back to work. That brings us to a real-world conundrum: motherhood, nursing, and work.

THE CULTURAL DILEMMA

Half of new mothers are back at work within the first year of an infant's life—and the majority of that half are on the job by the time the baby is three months old.[12] Breast milk is the best choice for feeding infants because of its perfect mix of nutrients; because it brings mother and baby into intimate, soothing contact; and because of its association with some health benefits. Here's where societal mixed messages come in. As noted earlier, the American Academy of Pediatrics, in its 2005 policy statement, recommends breast feeding exclusively for six months.[13] No formula supplements. No cereal. Just mother's milk. It further recommends continuing breast feeding for a year while introducing other foods. Only 15 percent of new mothers follow that recommendation,[14] leaving 85 percent of mothers with yet another reason to feel guilty or inadequate.

Yet while urging women to nurse for up to a year, our society also says, "Don't expect any help from us." Many new mothers want to or must get back to work. In a study of 173 countries, the United States was one of only four countries—along with Liberia, Papua New Guinea, and Swaziland—without any provision for paid maternity leave.[15]

Federal law requires that women receive twelve weeks of *unpaid* maternity leave after giving birth, with assurance that they will get their old jobs back when they return.[16] But the federal law has loopholes. People have to have been on the job for at least a year, and the law does not apply to part-time workers or to small employers of fifty or fewer people. That leaves a lot of workers unprotected. And it leaves all workers without a guarantee of income during their leave. Only 16 percent of companies with one hundred or more employees provide full pay during maternity leave.[17]

Even the best of family-friendly companies, as chosen each year by the Institute for Women's Policy Research, found that among their one hundred top-rated companies, about a quarter provided four weeks or fewer of paid maternity leave. And half of those companies—the beacons of hope for mothers and fathers who want time with their newborns—offer no paternity or adoption leave whatsoever.[18]

Most women, if they want three months at home with their newborn, stitch together a patchwork of unused vacation time and sick days, then are left crossing their fingers that they don't need another sick day any time during the next year. (In five states, California, Hawaii, New Jersey, New York, and Rhode

Island, new mothers can collect temporary disability payments.) In the United States, only 7 percent of women are back at work when their infant is one month old. But at two months, a quarter of new mothers are back at work, and by the time the infant is three months old, 41 percent of mothers are back on the job. Some 60 percent of women with babies nine months or younger are working.[19]

And once women are back at work, few companies offer on-site or nearby day care so that these women can dash out during the day to nurse their infants. More often, babies of working mothers who want to continue breast feeding are no longer literally breast-fed while their mothers are gone. Rather, they are fed expressed breast milk out of a bottle, kept fresh in the refrigerator or freezer and then reheated. For working women who can close their office door, afford a state-of-the-art breast pump, and maintain some control over their work schedule, pumping is possible, but it's also time-consuming and difficult. For women whose workplace bathroom is a pit or who have to wolf down their sandwich while pumping, it can be a near-impossible challenge to express an adequate supply of breast milk. With expressed milk, a father or a nanny or a grandmother or a day care worker holds the bottle. The container is now indistinguishable from a formula bottle.

In order to follow the AAP guidelines, many women have to figure out a way to still feed their babies maternal milk when they must leave them.

BREAST PUMPS AND FROZEN MILK

The reality of life in America has set the stage for a study that would have had our grandmothers scratching their heads. Breast milk stored in the refrigerator at thirty-nine degrees Fahrenheit keeps its nutritional value, and remains safe from bacteria, for at least four days.[20] Who knew? It should be stored in a clean, dry, glass container or a plastic container free of the chemical bisphenol A, which is suspected of adversely affecting children's development. Freezing breast milk can result in the destruction of some infection-fighting cells and also minimally reduces its nutritional value.

What nobody knows is whether pumping and freezing breast milk and having it delivered in a bottle by a father or a nanny offers the same benefit as breast milk coming directly from the source. A whopping 85 percent of breast-feeding mothers pump and store their milk at some point during the time they're breast-feeding.[21] Some nutritionists, like Kathleen Rasmussen at Cornell University, urge more study on the consequences—good and bad—of expressing breast milk and feeding it to infants from bottles. For now, she argues, not enough is known about whether and how much nutritional content is diminished by collecting, storing, and thawing the milk.

Whatever is in the bottle, and whoever is doing the feeding, the process should come as close to the feel of breast feeding as possible. That means holding and cuddling the infant, looking into her eyes, kissing her forehead, stroking her cheek, letting her bare skin touch parts of an adult's bare skin, whether chest or arm.

Adoptive mothers and working mothers can find breast feeding impossible or very difficult. Blasphemous as it may sound, some women are turned off by putting an infant to their breast. And for still others, the process is so painful and troublesome that they turn to formula as a logical alternative, concluding that it's better for their own circumstances. They remain excellent mothers, fostering closeness and bonding during feeding and taking advantage of decades of nutritional research in developing formulas.

THE SECRET SOCIETY
OF NONBREAST FEEDERS

Sandy LeBan of Wheaton, Illinois, wanted to nurse her daughter Natalie, but it didn't work out. She had a difficult labor that ultimately resulted in a cesarean delivery. But before Natalie arrived, Sandy had pushed so hard that every muscle in her body was sore—her arm muscles were so worn out she couldn't even hold her newborn. Swollen all over, she couldn't nurse for a few days. Sandy's mother would hold and feed Natalie while Sandy hooked herself up to a breast pump. Nothing was coming out. "I was in pain, miserable, and I had two suction cups on my boobs," she says. "I was dry as dry can be." A lactation specialist told her to keep it up.

Her last night in the hospital, she looked at those suction cups and swore off. "I thought, I'm torturing myself, I'm not able to feed her. This is just ridiculous," she says.

Throughout her ordeal, the hospital television was tuned to the baby channel. What sounded to her like scolding voices were telling her she *should* breast-feed. The gist of what she heard, as held in her memory, is no doubt more severe than the actual words: "If you don't nurse, you're the most awful mother in the world. Your baby will be deficient."

Her husband, Frank, made it clear he'd support any decision she made. "Hey, we were all Similac babies, and we're fine," he said. "You're not a bad person. You're a wonderful mother."

She went home and formula-fed. In so doing, she felt she joined what she called the "Secret Society of Nonbreast Feeders." Early on, she met another new mother with a bottle in her hand. Slowly, they risked admitting to each other that the liquid in the bottle was formula. They compared notes, listing the things they liked about formula feeding: Husbands can do some night feedings. Mothers get to sleep a little more at night, and they don't have to worry about getting infected nipples.

"I'm not knocking anyone who can do it," says Sandy. "In fact, I'm a little jealous of ladies who can nurse easily. But you shouldn't feel like you have to hide in a closet if you're a formula feeder."

FORMULA: THE NEXT BEST THING

Formula has come a long way since Dr. Benjamin Spock's recipe—evaporated milk plus sugar—appeared in his original *Common Sense Book of Baby and Child Care*, which came out in 1946. Formulas now contain necessary energy-providing nutrients (protein, carbohydrate, and fat), water, vitamins, and minerals. Whenever new information comes out on the specific nutrients found in breast milk, formula manufacturers attempt to keep up. Today, standard baby formulas are nutritionally complete, though breast milk no doubt contains additional as-yet-undiscovered and unstudied micronutrients.

The newest additions to some formulas since 2002 are docosahexaenoic acid (DHA) and arachidonic acid (ARA), two nutritional fatty acids considered building blocks for brain development and eye tissue. Some researchers believe that they are responsible for those few added IQ points in breast-fed babies.[22]

The American Academy of Pediatrics has not taken a stand on formulas with the new additions, which cost about 15 percent more than formulas without DHA and ARA. Study results are mixed regarding whether these truly benefit either cognitive development or vision, and current studies show no evidence of harm from the added ingredients. Pediatricians are the best source of information about the formula that's best for an individual baby.

BABIES WILL LOVE
THE FOODS THEIR PARENTS LOVE

There's an institute in—where else?—France called the European Center for Taste Science, which has shown that babies develop a taste for certain foods, and a disinterest in others, even in utero. In 2001, researchers at the center showed for the first time that newborn infants respond to foods their mothers have consumed.[23] The researchers used anise, a strong, licorice-flavored spice, as a test. Infants born to mothers who had consumed anise during pregnancy turned toward the smell of anise as newborns; infants whose mothers had not eaten anise turned away. Amniotic fluid can smell of cumin, garlic, onion, or other strong odors, and new research suggests that the fluid, as it passes through the fetus's oral and nasal cavities, may be laying the groundwork for future taste preferences.

Taste can be further influenced by what a lactating mother eats after her baby is born. The future taste preferences of formula-fed as well as breast-fed babies, research shows, is influenced by the cooking odors that fill the house. So steam those beets and broccoli florets, bake some halibut, throw some blueberries in those muffins, and cook up a nice pot of tomato basil pasta. Better yet, have a friend do it. Enjoy, and let the baby take in the aroma of good health.

BREAST FEEDING AND MOM'S HEALTH

I still remember, forty years later, the peace and quiet of breast feeding. Some women want the freedom to breast-feed in malls, restaurants, or other public places without the judgment of onlookers. I sympathize with that desire, but it was never my personal choice to breast-feed in public. I loved the opportunity to break away from a family gathering or a group of friends, take my baby into a quiet room, and have time alone, just the two of us. I think I enjoyed that solitude as much as anything else about nursing.

But there are other benefits. The uterus contracts faster, returning to prebirth size in less time than it does in formula-feeding mothers. Nursing delays the return of ovulation as long as a woman breast-feeds exclusively. But beware. It's not fail-safe birth control, so talk to an obstetrician about birth control choices while breast-feeding.

Breast feeding burns extra calories, though many women will say this benefit is offset somewhat by a voracious appetite while nursing. The average woman is about three pounds heavier six months after giving birth than she was before she got pregnant, and up to one woman in five is at least eleven pounds heavier six months after the birth. When researchers examined multiple studies on the relationship between breast feeding and future weight, they found a negligible difference—less than two pounds at a year to two years after birth—with breast-feeding mothers weighing slightly less than formula-feeding mothers.[24]

The same analysis found no long-term reduction in osteoporosis among older women who had breast-fed decades earlier. Just imagine all the possible variables—diet, exercise, smoking—between breast-feeding in one's twenties or thirties and developing osteoporosis in one's seventies or eighties!

The news is better when it comes to helping to prevent adult-onset diabetes, postpartum depression, breast cancer, and ovarian cancer. Studies have found an *association* between breast feeding and a future reduction—though very slight—in the risk of those diseases.

The reduction in risk for all the diseases studied was nil or small; and of the hundreds of studies involving hundreds of thousands of women, the differences in age, race, income, dietary habits, and countless other variables are incalculable. Breast feeding might improve women's health, but other lifestyle habits are far more likely to be of benefit. Good diet and exercise are measures known to improve health and quality of life.

RISK REDUCTION
ISN'T RISK ELIMINATION

Doing all the right things doesn't mean you won't be blindsided by disease. My sister, Nancy, had her first child at the age of twenty-one. She had three additional children before she was thirty, and she breast-fed all of them. Having children at a young age and breast-feeding them was supposed to protect her, she learned years later, from certain cancers, including ovarian cancer. But that was not her reason for having babies or for nursing them. She did it because she wanted to.

Thank goodness for that, because those measures didn't protect her. She was diagnosed with ovarian cancer at the age of fifty-eight, and a cruel eighteen months later she died. In the interim, she found out that she did not have the BRCA gene, which greatly increases the risk of both ovarian and breast cancer. She had no family history of ovarian cancer; this horrible disease came out of nowhere. There was no predicting she'd get ovarian cancer—and no stopping it when it arrived.

I'm glad she had her babies young, because she lived to see four children go to college, develop careers, get married, and produce nine grandchildren. She lived long enough to blossom with pride when her oldest grandson won a football scholarship to Purdue University. Her family was the center of her universe, and she loved her life. I'm glad she breast-fed her infants, because she enjoyed every minute of it. I'm also glad she didn't breast-feed under the mistaken expectation that it would miraculously protect her from future harm.

As women ponder their feeding choices, one question that can be answered only by individual women is this: what's better for baby—breast milk or a happy mother? Loving the experience of breast feeding should be the reason for doing it. A baby will be content with a happy, attentive mother whether she's offering a breast or holding a bottle.

CHAPTER FIVE

Sound

Laying the Foundation for Speech

A fire truck screaming, a vacuum cleaner roaring, a talk show host droning, grown-ups chattering, children nattering, dishes clattering. For a newborn baby, the sounds are all there, but the brain isn't ready to assign more or less importance to any one of them. As a fetus, he heard most of it before, but in utero the sounds were mercifully muffled, almost soothing. The most soothing of all sounds in the new world no doubt is also the most familiar—mother's voice, a crucial comfort as the newborn enters his new world. Newborns recognize their mothers' voices, turning toward them more readily than toward any other voices from the moment of birth. But they'll quickly respond to consistently present new voices, like those of adoptive parents.

Hearing is the most highly developed sense at birth—but a newborn cannot yet discern what is worth listening to and what can be safely ignored. Imagine hearing a dog bark before knowing what a dog is. Now imagine the dog barking, the television set blaring, and an older sister crying.

To understand what a newborn is going through, imagine being in a foreign country for the first time. There are endless strange and wonderful sights and sounds assaulting your senses simultaneously. But you can't read the street signs, you don't understand what people are saying, and the aromas from restaurants are strange. "You want to know what it's like to be a baby?" says Dr. Alison Gopnik, professor of psychology at the University of California, Berkeley, to an audience of child development workers. "It's like being in love for the first time in Paris after four double espressos. It's fantastic. It's a wonderful state to be in. And very likely, you'll wake up at three A.M. . . . *crying.*"[1]

FIRST SOUNDS

Newborns cannot at first sort through the din. But quickly, over the first three months, an infant will develop the ability to organize sounds. She does it bit by bit, building up an internal representation of her world. During the fourth trimester, a baby's brain is soaking up sounds, being bathed in the acoustics of her surroundings. It's a passive exposure that no one can see, but the sounds are sculpting the very brain circuits that will soon allow her to figure out where one word ends and another begins. It's the foundation she'll use to later form her own syllables, words, and sentences and to connect words to people, things, and activities.

In the first few weeks, an infant is capable of making only a narrow range of sounds, and those are largely outbursts: a cry, a hiccup, a burp, a sneeze. But even those are teaching him the art of communication. He's noticing that his mother pays attention to each sound, offering comfort, a laugh, a rub, or a startled look accompanied by "gesundheit." His noise, he's figuring out, gets a response. Sometime around two months, the baby will start cooing. As he leans back, his tongue may hit the roof of his mouth, the perfect position for uttering the hard *g* or *k* sound. He may decide to follow it with the easiest vowel sound for him to utter—*oo*. Infants with parents who coo back, or even silently smile or tenderly touch them, soon babble more than infants whose cooing is ignored. The enthusiasm of the response will only encourage him to try again and again.

WHAT WE HAVE
LEARNED FROM SONGBIRDS

Human infants would never learn to speak if they didn't hear adults teach them by example. It's the same for birds. Songbirds learn their unique tune the same way humans learn to speak: by imitation.

Among zebra finches, for example, singing the species' song is exclusively a male activity, so the father is in charge of teaching it. Scientists have observed male mentors taking over for an absent father songbird, but it's important that the teaching relationship is one on one—the same kind of devoted attention every baby needs. Until they're about twenty-five days old, both male and female zebra finches cheep and peep, but they haven't developed their distinctive song yet. Within the next five days, there's a dramatic development in the males: a pathway develops between two parts of the brain that are thought to be similar to speech-control areas in both male and female human brains. But the pathway, prompted by male hormones, never develops in the female zebra finch brain. The females continue to chirp and cheep but never learn the family song. Meanwhile, the males' song gets progressively louder. They try out a lot of vocalizations and gradually a pattern emerges.[2]

Like a human baby, the infant zebra finch appears to begin to absorb the elements of the language he'll need from birth, before he utters any of his own sounds. He starts in the same way that human infants begin—by listening. By thirty-five days of age, the young songbird is starting to imitate his father's song, or that of an attentive male mentor, but he doesn't yet have it quite right. It's something akin to baby babbling. But by three months of age, the male zebra finch is singing the song passed down through generations. It's a tune he'll repeat for the rest of his life, and when the time comes he'll pass it on exactly as he learned it to his own infant sons.

Baby birds alone in captivity don't learn to sing from a recording of an adult songbird. Just like human infants, they need the individual attention of an adult who cares. A tape recorder or a television set simply isn't good enough. They need the give and take of social interaction.

HOW INFANTS LEARN LANGUAGE

It's miraculous and mysterious that infants go from hearing a cacophony of sounds to recognizing that words are distinct from woofs, meows, and clanging pots and pans. Furthermore, from the flood of words they hear strung together, they have to figure out where one word ends and another begins. All of this is going on long before they babble or utter their own first words. We all sense that important things are happening in that brain as we ponder: "I wonder what he's thinking."

Some of a baby's potential for learning is no doubt factory installed, present within the wiring of the brain at birth.

Infants can't learn without some inborn capabilities. But they also can't learn without real-life experience—a combination of both nature and nurture. "Science is now putting these two philosophies together," says psychologist Dr. Jenny Saffran, director of the Infant Learning Laboratory at the University of Wisconsin-Madison. "It's an incredibly rich world, and infants have a toolkit to make sense of it."[3] Learning is the bridge between what's in the brain at birth and the fascinating world outside.

Babies around the world are born capable of hearing all sound distinctions uttered in the entire human race's various languages. They're capable of hearing the ones that will become part of their native language, as well as others they may never need as they grow up. This universal inborn ability to hear and differentiate the sounds in all human language is soon lost—pruned away by a brain that has learned early on that it won't need to make the sound distinctions not used in the homeland.

Dr. Patricia Kuhl, a neuroscientist and professor of speech and hearing at the University of Washington and a leading expert on speech development, has done groundbreaking work on this subject. Working with very young infants in Japan, she discovered why it is that Japanese people have difficulty mastering the *ra* and *la* syllables of the English language. Dr. Kuhl and her colleagues tested infants using special pacifiers connected to computers. The infants loved new sounds, and sucked up to eighty times a minute to keep the sound going.[4] Think of Maggie Simpson sucking like mad when aroused by the antics of her cartoon father, Homer. But infants, like all of us, get bored with repetition. They eventually slowed down after hearing the same sound over and over. Then as a new sound was introduced, they again sped up their sucking.

Using these special pacifiers, researchers found that infants as young as one month of age heard all sound distinctions—the ones that would become part of their native language, as well as others that they were unlikely to hear as adults. The Japanese babies in the study could tell there was a change in sound when they heard *rake* and then *lake*. Japanese adults cannot make the distinction—even the Japanese scientists involved in the experiment couldn't do it.

Kuhl found that at seven months of age, Japanese babies could still discriminate between the *ra* and the *la* sounds. But when tested just three months later, at ten months of age, the babies could no longer make the distinction. If they heard the *ra* sound long enough to get bored, and then the sound changed to *la*, they remained bored and inattentive. Whatever inborn ability they had to make the distinction was lost to brains that were preparing themselves for the sounds that would be needed in the Japanese babies' native land.[5]

And so it is around the world. A French baby and an American baby have the same ability, for around a half a year, to hear the guttural, rolling *r* of the French language. Within ten months, the American baby has lost it, and if she tries to learn the French language as a teen or an adult, the unnatural attempt to say *rouge* or *après* can be challenging, if not downright embarrassing.

MOZART, MUSIC, AND RHYTHM

The trend to expose infants and older babies to Mozart and other classical music has taken off. Surely, it can't be bad. But there's no one type of music that is better for development than any other. Dr. Russell Hamer, a sensory scientist at the University of São Paulo in Brazil is affiliated with the Smith-Kettlewell

Eye Research Institute, San Francisco. Though he specializes not in hearing but in infant vision, he is around babies a lot in research settings. He offers this bit of wisdom about the sounds in a child's world:

> It is probably good to expose your baby to a range of music and rhythms, including folk music from around the world—not just Mozart, not just any one kind of music. Rhythm is such a basic experience and surely goes back in human history before the evolution of full language. It is in the heartbeat, the gait of one's own body, the breath, the changes of light and dark, sun and moon, waves on a beach, the sounds of animal feet and bird's wings. Song and musical tones are also surely ancient experiences and deep in our communicative past. Melody and harmony live inside our own vocalizations.[6]

The rhythms of the natural world, along with the music of the masters and a dose of family favorites—rock and roll, jazz, blues, or country—will give an infant the opportunity to start bopping to the beat.

FROM SOUNDS TO SYLLABLES

The sounds from the voices she's hearing are forming patterns that are her first exercise in math. With an innate skill that would make a statistics student jealous, she's keeping track of probabilities. Her brain is noting the language she hears, setting up neural connections in response to the probability of a sound occurring, of it pairing with a preceding sound, or of it following another sound.

Infants even a few weeks old can pull apart the ingredients of language. We know, for example, that they can tell the difference between the sounds *pa* and *ba*. How did we discover this? Again, by testing infants using computers connected to that old standby, the pacifier. When the infants heard a new sound *(pa)* their sucking rate increased; when they'd had enough, their sucking slowed. Then, when a new and different sound was introduced *(ba)* they were once again intrigued and their sucking sped up again.[7]

There's a lot going on in that head in the first few months, which we don't yet know enough about to measure. But by about six months of age, babies have developed strategies for figuring out where one word ends and another begins. While younger infants have not been studied for their ability to recognize word boundaries, we can assume that, from birth, infants are stockpiling an arsenal of sounds. During the fourth trimester, they are laying the groundwork to parse syllables, figuring out which ones belong within a word and which ones begin the next word.

Here's an example. How many times have you cooed *pretty* and paired it with *baby* during the infant's first weeks and months? A lot, I'd guess. But sometimes you deviate. A mother might call her a pretty girl, or him a pretty boy. Or a father or grandparent might be even more specific: *Pretty Maggie. Pretty Brian.* The infant is learning that the syllables in *pretty—pret* and *ty—*go together fairly reliably. But every now and then, that combination of sounds—*pret-ty—*is followed by *baby* or *girl* or *boy* or a name. Hearing the word *pretty* over and over reliably informs the baby that those two sounds go together, that they form a word. Hearing it paired with a few different sounds, *baby,* or *boy,* or *girl,* teaches the infant that the word *pretty* stands by itself and is separate from the other words that may follow. Using the law of probability, infants are learning which syllables are likely to occur together.

We do the same thing as adults listening to a foreign language. When words are spoken quickly, it's difficult to hear where one ends and another begins. For a baby, her own native language is a foreign language at first, and her brain is soaking it all up, filing it away in brand-new neural connections for a lifetime of future use. She is quietly but consistently taking note of the sounds, long before she utters her first *da-da* or *ma-ma*.

Background noise can be a distraction for an infant, just as it is for adults. In the uterus, noise was muffled. During this time of transition, it's important to give infants some time to hear only a single voice, with background noise minimized. It wasn't so for our ancient ancestors struggling for survival in, say, the Serengeti of eastern Africa. Then, listening to the broadband overview of noise helped with survival. But today's clatter of television sets and radios can hinder an infant's ability to learn the tones and sounds that make up language, so take time regularly to read or speak to infants with as few background distractions as possible.[8] Middle-of-the-night feedings can be good for such quiet, intimate encounters.

WHEN HEARING IS BLOCKED

We know from kitten studies (this is discussed in chapter 6) that temporarily blocking vision in infancy affects the brain's wiring. Only recently have scientists, led by researchers at the Massachusetts Eye and Ear Infirmary, learned that short-term hearing problems, such as an ear infection that blocks sound in one ear, can also affect the brain's initial wiring in its hearing centers. The blockages can cause problems long after the infection is cleared up.[9]

So far, we know this only from animal studies. Experimenting with newborn rats, scientists blocked hearing in one ear and then examined the rats' brains. They found that the neural connections in centers of the brain involved in sound from that ear were weakened, while those connections getting input from the normal ear were strengthened.

When results of this work were published, Dr. Daniel Polley, the lead researcher from Massachusetts Eye and Ear Infirmary, said he received many email messages from adults who remembered having a lot of ear infections as children. "There was a groundswell," he says. "I heard from people who had ear infections as kids and felt they could never participate fully in the fast moving language of the world."[10] They reported difficulty in following conversation when more than one person was speaking, or trouble hearing well in, say, a crowded restaurant, where tableside conversation competes with a lot of background noise.

The outlook, however, is better for those who experience temporarily blocked hearing in infancy than it is for those who undergo blocked vision, which can result in permanent vision loss. As soon as the ear infection clears and normal hearing is restored, the brain begins setting up those connections it missed forming earlier, though scientists still don't know if hearing is eventually fully restored to normal. And since ear infections are the number one reason that parents take their children to pediatricians, it's important to study the effect of temporary sound distortion caused by infections.

While there's still a lot to study concerning the long-term effects of early ear infections, Polley says that such infections come and go, and the brain can make good use of even short periods of good, clean sound input. "Even with chronic and persistent ear infections, there's good reason to believe that through [later] training with a speech pathologist, [children] can recover normal hearing and speech."

BILINGUAL BABIES

The world seems to be getting smaller, and in the United States about 20 percent of children live with at least one foreign-born parent. Add in the numbers of infants cared for by non-English-speaking nannies or other non-English-speaking caregivers, and that's a lot of babies hearing more than one language from the day they're born.

Scientists once thought that learning two languages simultaneously was confusing for an infant and might slow down her ability to learn one language well. That notion has been proven false. It's no harder for a baby to learn two languages than it is to learn one. Speak regularly in both, and, far from becoming confused, she will learn to say her first word right on developmental schedule, at about a year. And about six months after that, she'll have a vocabulary of approximately fifty words, just like her monolingual peers. Research shows that some motor skills of bilingual infants may even be slightly better, and that these infants may have a better ability to pay attention. That could be because they've had practice in listening to one language while not allowing knowledge of the other to interfere. They've gained the skill of paying attention to the language being spoken while keeping the other language temporarily on hold.[11] It's important, though, to keep the languages separate. Don't throw an English word or phrase into a Spanish sentence, or vice versa.

There are certainly advantages for the child who speaks more than one language. He'll feel at home among his peers at school as well as among family members who might be more comfortable with their native tongue. And when he's old enough to be launched into the working world, his bilingualism may be the deciding factor in landing a good job!

But don't go crazy and take an immersion course in Swedish so that the baby will learn two languages. Parents are not depriving their babies if they speak only one language. Babies are remarkably prepared to accept whatever home they're born into, and keeping things natural is the best way to prepare a newborn for the life she's got.

ADOPTED BABIES
AND NEW PARENTS' VOICES

Adopted babies may need a bit more time to identify their mothers' voices, but they do catch up. Beth Wheeler and her partner, Emmy, adopted a son, Matai, when he was a month old. Beth recalls the frustrating strangeness of their first meeting. She also well remembers the joy of infant-maternal "conversation" just two weeks later. Matai had spent his first weeks with a nurturing foster mother, and it was clear he had already learned to love her voice, even though it wasn't the one he heard in the womb. "He was very comfortable with her, familiar with her," says Wheeler. "She would speak, and you could see there was a slight movement from him toward her voice. He kind of melted into her arms." But during that initial meeting, when Beth spoke to their new baby there was no such response. "When she handed him to us, he fidgeted, like he was trying to get used to something he didn't know," she said.

Then, when Matai was two months old, it all changed. He moved toward his new parents' voices, locked into their eyes, responded to their touch. By three months of age, he would coo and gurgle in conversational response to his adoptive parents' words. "It's like we're talking to each other. He feels heard. We feel heard. When we're playful with him, he makes all sorts of sounds," says Wheeler. No doubt, he was paying attention to his foster mother's voice during his first few weeks. But soon his allegiance switched. It may take a bit longer, but with lots of talking and other sounds from parents, adopted babies come to recognize the sound of familiar, loving voices.

What any baby needs is a devoted connection, and he'll find it where it's offered: from mother or father—whether biological or adoptive—caregiver, or grandparent. He's prepared to tune in to those who love him, and his devotion to a loving, responsive voice only enhances each parent's natural desire to communicate more.

THE LANGUAGE OF PARENTESE

Just look at a baby when speaking to her, and see how intently she listens. She's storing what she's hearing, taking note of patterns of sounds that are an important initial step in her language development. So talk to her. Tell her about your day. Ask her about hers. None of it has to make logical sense. As she sits on the kitchen table in her infant seat watching you unpack groceries, mention that the milk goes in the fridge and the cereal goes in the pantry. She'll be fascinated by such mundane conversation. Give her a tour of her new home, pointing out pictures, toys, even the washing machine. Those who babble like this are not talking to themselves. No doubt someone speaking to an infant will find himself speaking in rhythms and tones different from those used with other adults. But the words themselves are letting the baby know which sounds are going to be important, and she loves their resonance.

An infant will pay especially close attention to anyone, even someone he's never heard before, if words are spoken in, dare I say it, "baby talk." In fact, the high inflection adults use when speaking to him makes his ears perk up.[12] The term *baby talk* has nothing to do with actual word choices, like *toi-toi* instead of *toilet,* or *tum-tum* instead of *stomach.* Rather, it refers to a particular kind of voice that babies universally enjoy. Researchers used to call the voice "motherese," but now it's called "parentese" and could just as well be called "caretakerese" because almost all those who care for infants will find themselves speaking it: grandparents, aunts, uncles, babysitters, and just about everyone else. Whether in English, German, or Mandarin Chinese, people around the world use parentese. And the rhythm and intonation of the language that adults automatically use when speaking to infants help set the brain up to recognize where one word ends and another begins and to start constructing the appropriate synapses.[13] High-pitched and singsongy with notable pitch changes, the language babies love uses exaggerated vowels, short simple sentences, and a slower rhythm. It is usually accompanied by embellished facial expressions. Adults can hardly help it. They look at that cute bundle and go gaga.

And it's just what babies need as they begin to pick words out of the blur of fluent speech. The use of parentese makes the sounds of vowels more distinct from one another and produces expanded vowel sounds not found in ordinary adult conversations. (What a pretteee baaabeee.) This exaggerated dialogue helps a baby's brain analyze speech even before her mouth and vocal tract can form the sounds.

Right about now is a good time for the kind of advice that runs throughout these pages. Don't worry. Don't spend a second's worth of effort to elongate vowels or emphasize syllables. It'll come naturally. Each baby is busy laying down a network of communication synapses—increasingly elaborate connections within her brain, all enhanced by experience. And she's doing it automatically. Babies don't just sit there and wait for formal lessons. From day one, they recognize familiar sounds, like a parent's voice. And they're geared up to pay attention to unfamiliar sounds. Infants are busy making these distinctions long before they ever speak. They're listening, listening, listening. They're picking up on intonations. They're adjusting their very wails of life to what they're hearing in their native languages. The intonations of the cry of a German baby, after just a few days, differ from those of the cry of a French or American baby.

Baby-specific speech comes naturally to adults and ends up providing infants with essential nuggets of information about the language they'll soon be speaking. It's universal and will come so automatically that no one needs to worry about learning the language of parentese. People, using the patterns and rhythms of their native languages, do it in the United States, in Europe, in Asia, and in Africa—around the world.

By two months of age, a baby might begin to take turns in the conversation. He doesn't have much to say yet, of course. But he'll wait, stay quiet while a parent or caretaker speaks, then make noise when things turn quiet. He'll look intently at the adult's face as he makes sounds. He wants a response. Talk to him. Then listen for his response. Then speak again. It's better yet to look at him when speaking so he can connect facial expressions and emotions to words. Take advantage of this brief period of time when no words are boring or mundane, when every utterance is fascinating to at least one listener.

CHAPTER SIX

Sight

From Forms to Faces

From the moment of birth, a new baby is a visual feast. Relieved mothers and fathers count fingers and toes. Adoptive parents make the same fascinating full-body exam the minute they get the chance. They study the fine, downy hair on his head and, yes, on his ears and his back. They delight in the folds in his thighs, in his chubby cheeks, in his seeming lack of a neck. And if he deigns to gaze in their direction, they don't really care if he sees clearly or not. They're captivated. Adults will do any number of silly things to capture a second's glance: blow bubbles, exaggerate a smile, babble ridiculous sounds, or bore their own wide-eyed stare directly into his eyes.

The very act of opening his eyes is a little trick, one of many irresistible manipulations nature has provided that provoke a caretaking response. "A baby opens up his eyes and looks. It's a very powerful turn on," says Dr. Penny Glass, director of the Child Development Program at the Children's National Medical Center in Washington, D.C. "You think the baby is looking right smack dab at you."[1] It doesn't even matter that he doesn't see the details of the face that holds his attention, because every parent loves looking into the eyes of a new baby while trying to imagine the world from his point of view. And as parents gaze, they no doubt wonder: What is this brand-new being seeing when he looks back?

We know that vision is the least-developed sense at birth. Infants arrive able to recognize their mothers' voices, for example, but with no such ability to see or recognize her face. Yet they can discern shadows of eyes, edges of faces, and areas of high contrast. What they need in order to develop this complex sense during the fourth trimester is practice at "seeing." Each new flicker of vision establishes new neural connections that will eventually enable them to see. The slowly developing sense of vision, with its multiple components of focus, contrast, three-dimensionality, and color, will, during this time of transition, carry the infant from a world of darkness into the rich world of light.

What a baby sees is largely a mystery, even to science. Discerning what the world looks like to an infant is not as simple as, say, imagining a blurry video image slowly coming into focus. Infant vision no doubt has some elements of gradually increasing clarity over the first months. But since specific parts of the eye and the brain have to develop and coordinate during the fourth trimester in order for a view of the world to begin to make sense, we can only imagine what an infant's new world looks like.

But imagining her world is really not so hard. In fact, it's exactly what parents have been doing for millions of years— imagining what their baby sees. What science does know is that she wants to look, she wants to see, and she seeks out the edges of our faces, the shadows of our eyes, as her very first exploration. That initial and nearly sightless exploration actually begins to build columns of neural connections that will ensure her good vision as she grows.

THE EDGES OF A BABY'S WORLD

Conventional wisdom holds that a newborn sees almost nothing, but parents know better. In their earliest observations, mothers, fathers, caregivers, and physicians recognize that an infant is connecting to the world with his eyes. His vision is the least mature of his senses at birth, but recent research shows that he's seeing more than anyone imagined even a decade ago. It begins with objects of high contrast and distinct edges.

One such object in the household of Frank and Sandy LeBan was a ceiling fan in the family room. A plain white globe below four brown blades, the fan presents a crisp contrast to the white ceiling above. Natalie LeBan was born on December 15, 2009, and arrived at her suburban Wheaton, Illinois, home during a typical Illinois winter. There was snow on the ground, and the city would soon be hit by its first arctic blast of the season. As the furnace kicked out bursts of heat, the fan's dark blades were still.

And yet, from the moment Natalie laid eyes on that ceiling fan she loved it, motionless and boring though it was. "When she's about to blow, the way to calm her is with the ceiling fan," Sandy said. It worked when she was just days old, and it still worked three months later as Sandy talked to me. "We stand under the fan. It doesn't move, but she gets mesmerized. She starts staring, and she gets calm."

"I think it's the contrast," said Frank.

He's exactly right, according to a body of research on how infant vision develops. "Infants are drawn to high contrast," says

T. Rowan Candy, associate professor of optometry and associate dean of research at Indiana University School of Optometry. "It takes a while to coordinate the movement of the eyes. For the first month or two, the eyes may not be fully aligned on the parents' faces. But they're drawn to high contrast."[2]

It's not just ceiling fans. Infants see the edges of a face, and know its shape and profile, long before they see the details that make our physiognomies unique.[3] The edge of a loving face is a baby's first lesson that objects occupy a finite space, that where a parent's face ends, the rest of the world begins. By paying attention to the borders of things, newborns begin to learn that the world is made up of separate, distinct objects.

When a newborn looks at mom's face, especially if there's bright light behind her head, he'll look at the side of the head rather than into the eyes. Equipped to learn more from the endless variety of expressions on a familiar face, seen at first as the shadows of eyes and mouth, an infant doesn't need the eye candy of toys. "Whatever you put around them, it shouldn't compete with your face," says Dr. Glass.

A mother's face, or that of a father or caretaker, is an infant's lifeline, and she likes it more than anything else she'll lay eyes on. Even ceiling fans are just a temporary distraction. She will soon recognize the face of one who loves her, and she won't make judgments about beauty. The natural impulse of parents, grandparents, and other loving adults is to feast their eyes—and that's exactly what babies need. They are, undoubtedly, feasting back.

SEEING THROUGH BABY'S EYES

Vision has multiple components—the ability to see detail, to be sensitive to gradations of light and dark, to distinguish colors and forms, to perceive depth and distance, and ultimately, to recognize objects and faces—all developing simultaneously and at different rates. A common belief is that newborns have a range of focus that goes roughly from mom's face to her breast. It's a pleasant, maternal myth, this notion that infants arrive able to see their mothers' faces—which are typically seven to ten inches away—while being fed. A lot of infant development books still refer to that estimated distance.

"This is a wonderful myth to debunk," says Dr. Russell Hamer, a sensory scientist at the University of São Paulo in Brazil who is affiliated with the Smith-Kettlewell Eye Research Institute, San Francisco. "That 'seven to ten inches' started in 1965 with one study by psychologist Robert Fantz. It's since been disproven, but it persists. It's just not true."[4] Fantz's contribution to infant developmental science was the creation of a way to measure an infant's looking behavior. The myth endures because infants do indeed look toward their mothers' faces when they're feeding. They can't yet notice details, however. What catches their eyes is the contrast between hairline and face, or between her profile and the wall behind, or the shadows of her eye sockets.

Infant vision is not nearly as good as normal adult vision, but that's not the whole problem. Infants also have trouble shifting their focus from near to far. Their best distance for viewing, for approximately the first month, is probably about a foot away; anything closer or farther away is blurred. So a newborn may be most fascinated by, say, a hairline. That'll change in about a month, but at first it's borders and edges he's drawn to.

How infant vision is characterized is a matter of perspective—kind of a "glass half-empty" or "glass half-full" comparison based on two parallel streams of science. There's the modern version of Fantz's original behavioral testing, the "half-empty" way of looking at things. Now there are also findings from more recent research that provide a "glass half-full" perspective. New technology, called "visual evoked potential," measures aspects of vision using, say, flashing lights or video screen patterns, then looks for changes on an electroencephalograph.[5] It's this new way of looking for EEG changes—changes that indicate brain activity in response to lights or patterns—that makes researchers believe babies see more than we once thought.

THE FIRST MONTH

So what is a newborn baby seeing? We can't truly know. The technological measures available can look at elements of the eye and the brain. For example, scientists can observe that the lens is passively refracting light.[6] They can see muscles around the eye changing the shape of the lens. They can also watch a baby orient correctly to the sight of his mother's face. See table 2.

Science gives us clues about how the various aspects of infant vision are developing. For example, we know that a newborn can see the big *E* on an eye chart. That's pretty amazing, when you think about the size of that large *E*. It corresponds with things that are most important for an infant to see: fingers, faces, nipples, and their own toes. "Their vision is good enough to give a huge amount of information to a developing brain," says Hamer.[7]

An infant can look to the sky and focus on the full moon. In someone's arms, he looks toward shadowy areas of the face, like eyes, nose, lips, and teeth. He even seems to catch sight of his fingers when they cross his line of vision. Each of those aspects can be measured in research settings, but the sum of the findings still leaves us scratching our heads about what infants actually see.

TABLE 2
Vision Milestones

At Birth

- Infants can see poor but measurable contrast between very light and very dark objects. At a distance of one foot, they can see high-contrast black lines only 1/16″ wide on a white board.
- They can see movement of large, high-contrast objects.
- They can notice the edge of a face against a light background, although it is hazy, blurry, undefined, and bland.

One Month

- Infants can see some red and green, although colors aren't rich.
- They show some additional response to motions of large objects.
- They pay attention briefly to faces.

Two Months

- Infants have a growing visual palette that now includes more color.
- They are drawn to facial features, not just the edges of faces.
- They begin to respond to more subtle motions, like the movement of a hand in front of the baby's face.

Three Months

- Infants see color much better and more colors.
- They clearly notice movement and more often follow motion.
- They will kick and flail to hold the attention of people who make eye contact.
- A baby is likely to bring into his visual field an object, such as a rattle, that has been placed in his hand.
- Infants still have few clues for judging depth, but the haze is clearing.

SOURCE: Penny Glass, "What Do Babies See?" n.d., www.lighthouse.org/about-low-vision-blindness/childrens-vision/what-do-babies-see/, accessed May 9, 2010.

Newborns can follow a moving object with their eyes—if the object is large, has high contrast, and isn't moving too quickly. Just as edges and borders help them learn that objects are distinct from their backgrounds, movement also helps them learn the shapes of objects.[8] If the caregiver moves a bright yellow ducky with a black beak across a white blanket, the infant learns that the black and yellow bits are part of one moving object. The lesson is recorded as the brain creates new connections. During this time, his eyes will likely follow with a jerky motion, but he's learning what his toy looks like, and that it's a separate and distinct object.

Hamer, who has spent his career exploring infant vision, puts in perspective the difficulty of translating research findings into real-life understanding: "It has been a long, hard road for scientists trying to find clever ways of 'proving' even whether or not a baby can see black-and-white gratings, or trying to evaluate objectively what level of visual acuity a three-month-old, for example, has. Tracking, or following, eye movements does not tell you what aspects of the object being followed are actually perceived; nor does lack of following prove that an object was *not* perceived. It is a difficult business."[9]

While we await scientific proof, every parent knows instinctively that gazing into an infant's eyes is a deeply rooted, bonding form of communication. We do know that during the first month of life, a baby's vision is up to twenty times worse than an adult's best-corrected vision, according to behavioral studies. But move on to more modern visual-evoked-potential measures of vision, and the picture improves. Because of this technology, we realize that a newborn is seeing significant detail and, by one month of age, is seeing two to five times better than earlier, behavioral measures predicted.[10]

Imagine a high-quality Leica camera with a *great* lens. But the photographer chooses a grainy film. The fact that the final photo is of poor quality is no fault of the lens. And that's just one aspect of all the simultaneous and overlapping developments going on that add up to good vision.

At birth, the eyes, like the lens of a camera, work fairly well. Even as profound changes are occurring in the retina, the brain needs to mature and set up the neural connections necessary to develop the pictures. An infant can project a clean image onto the retina. But the part of the retina that gives good, detailed vision, called the fovea, is immature. When an infant looks at an object, the image projected onto the retina falls on a fovea too immature to transmit a clear image to visual areas of the brain. What we've got here, to borrow a line from the evil warden in the film *Cool Hand Luke,* is a failure to communicate. In time, and with the simple, inevitable practice of looking, the fovea will mature and the image transmitted will become clear.

In the first month of life, while babies can't distinguish between subtlely different shades of color, like red and orange, they can see large, colored patterns with a lot of contrast—say, dark blue against yellow.

None of this proves what babies see. And current behavioral studies still show that babies aren't responding in ways that let observers know they know what they're looking at. But information is making its way from the baby's eye to the developing visual centers of his brain.

MONTHS TWO AND THREE

In less than eight weeks, infants gain command of the muscles controlling, and the feedback systems guiding, the lens. By two months of age, they're looking deeper, staring intently at specific features—eyes, nose, and mouth. They love looking at our eyes, just as we love looking at theirs.

At two months, they might still be tracking movements with jerky eye motions, but by three months, their eye motions are becoming smoother. By this time, their attention is drawn to more subtle motion. A three-month-old infant might notice a fly landing on her father's nose.[11]

A similar story can be told about how babies process contrast. Studies show that, almost from birth, the brain is reliably signaling contrasts of objects—like Natalie LeBan's beloved fan blade against the ceiling. Sometime during the second month, sensitivity to contrast undergoes a huge burst in development, and infants can distinguish two shades of gray only slightly different from each other. By nine weeks to three months of age, they can see a white teddy bear on a white carpet. (Not that too many parents of newborns would invest in a white carpet.)

What they're seeing is changing their brains, establishing crucial neural connections that will affect their vision for their lifetimes. They still have a lot to learn. The lines of communication between the eye and the visual parts of the brain are undeveloped at first. But let's look at the "half-full" glass. Infants orient correctly. During the first three months, infants are shifting from responding to simple brightness or high-contrast edges (the outline of a face) to responding to organization of detail into a recognizable pattern (the eyes, a smile).

They love faces and they respond to movement. By two months, they're moving beyond mere light, movement, and high-contrast forms, and most will lock onto a human face, especially when the person is speaking. They'll be able to see some finer detail, more subtle contrast and shading.

An infant's eyes will soon move from the edges of a face and a hairline to an individual's eyes, nose, and mouth. He'll begin to notice changes, like eyes widening with delight or a mouth turning up into a smile. "They'll naturally seek out what is more complex," says Glass. "The face is very complex. They're watching for changes in facial expression. They soon develop a very sophisticated ability to respond to changes in facial expression. If you look away, it changes the baby's reaction and expression. We are human, so we're inherently social."

The picture continues to improve through the third month. Babies start watching people at a distance, and they can alternate between two people or objects. They'll start showing a preference for watching certain people, say, older brother over dad. Why not? He's more active and certainly sillier. By the end of the fourth trimester, count on the baby making out mother's eyes, father's smile, and her own small fingers and toes.

FIRST GLANCES

At birth, babies are already learning by looking. They learn most by watching those who most attentively watch them. "She watched my face almost from the beginning," Molly Lee said of her daughter, Abigail. "Scientifically, I know that's not valid."

Actually, scientifically, it *is* valid, despite the common wisdom that babies see nothing at birth. Abigail was surely watching the edge of her mother's face, not yet homing in on the eyes. So begins visual communication.

They're seeing—just not very clearly. In 1997, Dr. Davida Teller, a vision scientist and professor emerita at the University of Washington, Seattle, combined her wonder as a mother and grandmother and her expertise as a scientist to write *First Glances: The Vision of Infants.*

Newborns definitely see, she says. Their eyes catch the motion of large, high-contrast objects, like dad approaching a darkened room through a brightly lit doorway. Things may be hazy and blandly colored, but they're visible to a newborn. The natural environment provides exactly the amount of visual stimulation a baby needs. The animated images from everyday life begin to teach your baby about his world as they build his neural columns for lifelong sight.

SEEING DETAILS

What can babies really do? While even newborns can see a range of contrasts and sizes of objects, their focus is not yet accurate. "They can focus from infinity almost to the tip of their nose, right from birth," says Hamer. "But in the first few weeks, they don't have good control over the musculature that controls the shape of the lens, and hence the distance for which the eye is focused. They start being able to focus on different distances fairly accurately in two to three months. In parallel, during the first weeks and months, they are developing the coordination of their eye movements, an important part of the development of binocular vision."[12]

As children or adults, we can look at a television screen, and then a blank wall, and change optical focus quickly. But in order for that to happen, the circuitry that controls lens shape has to be in communication with the parts of the brain that analyze what we're seeing. It is the incoming visual information that "tells" the centers in the brain if an image is, or is not, in focus on the retina. For a baby to focus on an object, the muscles of the lens have to be in control, and newborns don't have that act coordinated. They can change focus pretty wildly in the first few weeks. Sometimes babies will go cross-eyed for a few moments from the effort. (If the problem of going cross-eyed persists beyond three months, consult a physician.)

An infant's lenses are much more pliable than an adult's. Throughout life, those lenses gradually get less and less pliable, leading to the inevitable presbyopia of middle age—and a need for reading glasses.

BRAIN NETWORKS

The brain sets up networks to bring baby out of the shadows. Getting from seeing light, movement, and forms to seeing actual faces takes important developmental work within the brain. The work starts in the uterus. It continues unobserved immediately after birth. The brain is busy sorting neurons and sending them to the proper brain regions, which are generating synapses so neurons can communicate. As those connections are formed, each baby gains an ability to make sense of what she's seeing. Neuroscientist Dr. Carla Schatz has likened those connections to a telephone system, where one line connects to a worldwide network.[13] Using chemical and electrical signaling, the brain is setting up networks of communication from brain cell to brain cell.

With about a million possible connections from each eye, lines of communication face a choice of about 2 million possible neural destinations. Ultimately, fewer than one hundred connections from eye to brain are actually selected. Those neural destinations that are chosen become permanent visual centers. Others that are not needed for vision or any other development wither away. But the ones that are used for connection complete the journey from the eye to the visual cortex in the back of the brain, transforming signals into sight. It is a daunting task.

So babies need to see in order to . . . well, continue to see. Visual experience completes the wiring.

THE HIGH COST OF VISUAL DEPRIVATION

If the visual pathways, ripe for development early in life, are completely blocked during crucial early periods, the result will be permanent visual impairment. But relax. A healthy baby living within anything resembling a normal human environment will not have those critical pathways blocked.

But children born with cataracts (a very rare condition), for example, have blocked visual pathways. If a child does not have the cataract removed to clarify vision within weeks of birth, she will remain visually impaired in the affected eye. Scientists have long known that there is some important visual wiring going on that must be done early, and that if it is not, then loss of vision in the brain may be permanent. Cataract surgery for adults is common and is almost always uneventful and successful at restoring vision. That's because adults have already had lifetimes of experience establishing visual centers in their brains.

Not so with infants. Using animal models in the 1960s, scientists sought to discover why children and adults have such different outcomes.[14] They discovered how the brain's visual cortex is organized, and how early experience in the world can change the organization. In experiments done with newborn kittens, they sewed shut one eye of each kitten and left it that way for several weeks. When the sutures were removed and the eye allowed to open, the kitten still could not see from that eye, even though the eye was perfectly normal. What the experiment showed was that if the eye and brain fail to make connections during crucial periods of development, the visual cortex undergoes dramatic reorganization and vision does not develop normally.

They repeated their work with monkeys. They found that in the normal monkey brain, there are columns of neurons in the visual cortex. Each column receives input from one eye, and the columns alternate between those dominated by information sent from the left eye and those dominated by information from the right eye. The alternating columns allow the brain to start putting that information together as binocular vision.

David Hubel and Torsten Wiesel, Nobel Prize–winning scientists who pioneered this vision work, found that, among the monkeys deprived of vision in one eye, the neural columns dominated by the seeing eye had in each case become wider. The neural columns that failed to receive input from the blinded eye had become narrower. It became clear that in order for monkeys or kittens to see normally, they had to have visual experiences during the earliest weeks or months of their lives. Without it, the brain's capacity to make the necessary neural connections was gone.

Hubel and Wiesel's research represents the best-studied example of how early experience affects the sculpting of the cortex during what scientists call critical periods. And this research led physicians in developed countries, including the United States and European countries, to provide urgently needed early treatment of, for example, babies born with congenital cataracts.

Unfortunately, in poor countries, where diagnosis and treatment are often unavailable, children with cataracts who don't receive medical attention until they are older are often not treated at all, because the medical world believes that even if vision is restored, the time for learning how to see has passed.[15]

MOBILES, FLASHING LIGHTS, AND BLACK-AND-WHITE TOYS

So what does all this talk of a critical period of visual development have to do with the majority of babies, who are born with every prospect for healthy vision?

A lot, it turns out. Parents are barraged with information—and misinformation—urging them to hurry up and make their babies smarter, happier, cuter, better, and to do it *right now*, before it's *too late*. Much of what parents are hearing is the source of unnecessary apprehension, anxiety, and guilt.

The blind-kitten and -monkey studies fed a lot of broad and unwarranted interpretations about learning and led to the urgency to do it right and do it immediately. Images of fast-growing neurons and withering neural connections within those tiny, immature brains entered American culture in a way that couldn't help but make parents nervous. The underlying assumptions based on neuroscience findings limited to vision in baby kittens and monkeys have made their way into an array of cultural beliefs that are not backed up by science.[16]

Remember, the blind-kitten and -monkey studies proved only that scientists could permanently destroy vision in kittens and monkeys by deliberately blocking their sight. This research, representing one of few hard neuroscience findings on infant development, also led to the proper conclusion that babies with conditions such as congenital cataracts must be treated early.

But misinterpretations and unwarranted leaps cover an astonishing range: from pressure to try teaching infants math and reading, to pressure to buy an array of toys and even infant clothing claiming to help individual babies become budding geniuses. If vision is withheld during a crucial period, the faulty thinking went, then what if multiplication tables are withheld? Or alphabet recognition? Such pressures are undoubtedly responsible for a heavy dose of parental guilt, even though the claims behind them don't hold water.

What followed those vision experiments was a remarkable leap in parental expectations and worries—not to mention marketers' claims. And then marketers made an additional leap. If deprivation was bad and stimulation was good, then more and more and more stimulation must be better. Buy this toy, they claimed, or that mobile—and for good measure, put a lot of blinking lights on everything. Or start teaching math and reading with flash cards as soon as babies open their eyes. There is not a shred of neuroscientific evidence to support such claims.

PERFECT VISUAL STIMULATION

The world provides perfect visual stimulation. Adding to parental pressure to hurry development along is another bit of misinterpreted scientific evidence. Vision researcher Davida Teller found that newborn babies responded strongly when presented with images of stark black-and-white stripes. Like Natalie LeBan, they were drawn to the contrast. Teller also found that babies had a weaker response when shown light-colored, or pastel, shades.

The result of these few bits of early vision science, combined with many unwarranted leaps to unjustified conclusions, became the perfect recipe for marketers' exaggerated claims. A new consumer trend was born: baby toys, clothes, and products in stark black and white.

"Black-and-white toys and mobiles," says Hamer. "That craze really took off, and every baby store had black-and-white clothing—everything. They were claiming it would promote your baby's brain development. They were marketing these things as if: 'If you don't use my toy, you might sacrifice brain development.' Babies *do* respond strongly to high contrast. It's built into the visual system. But it's fallacious to imply that if these high-contrast toys and things are not used, you'll be sacrificing normal visual development. The normal world is pretty rich. Literally millions of years of evolution have figured this out."[17] A ceiling fan provides high contrast. So do tree branches against a blue sky. So does a father's silhouette against the ceiling.

Modern parents, with nurseries, family rooms, and whole houses full of colorful, flashing toys, probably have more to fear from overstimulation than from understimulation. The normal environment—a parent's face, an aunt's dangling earring, or a basket balanced on an African woman's head—provides plenty of visual stimulation in even the poorest of circumstances. Don't worry about the colors in the mobile. Take the baby out to look at a tree.

If a newborn stares at a black-and-white mobile for a long time, who's to say that's a good thing? It may not be bad, but there's no evidence that it's either good or bad. "Consider the hypothesis that if they stare for a long time, you're visually trapping them," says Hamer. "I'm being melodramatic, but it's not that far-fetched."[18]

So don't worry. After all, in the uterus she was in the dark. Light and vision make their way slowly into her life during this time of transition. If a parent enjoys looking at something, her baby will like it. "Just think about our evolution in a natural environment, with people, faces, trees, birds, color, movement, rustling leaves, direct sunlight, dark clouds, black night," says Hamer. "We evolved in a *very* rich visual and multisensory environment."[19] So unless a home looks like a casino, or an infant is propped in front of the television for hours at a time or has nothing but a blank wall to stare at, people don't need to worry about visual overstimulation or understimulation. All he needs is love, parents and other caring adults, and the many unique things that make up a home.

SPEAKING WITH THEIR EYES

The conversation between parents and their newborn begins with faces and eyes. For Beth Wheeler, eye contact became a game. Her adopted son, Matai, had been born six weeks too early, and he was a month old when she adopted him. So when Matai was six weeks old—on what was supposed to be his arrival date—Wheeler saw a change. "Something happened. It was like he was born. His eyes shifted, seemed able to focus a little bit more. There had been almost a sense of vacancy in his eyes before that," she says. "Suddenly, it was like we could connect. Like there was a human there who could interact with another human."

With increased eye contact, Wheeler and Matai were off and running on their journey of love. Over the next few weeks, they began to have conversations—visual, eye-contact conversations. Then they added smiles and grimaces to the conversation. "We'd make facial expressions or smile. I'd widen my eyes. Then he'd do the same," she says. "Or if he was the one who started,

I'd mirror it. Then I knew: Okay, we're good to go. For a couple of months, he thrived on those visual conversations. He really talks through his eyes."

Yes, he does.

Infants as young as twelve days old imitate facial gestures.[20] "Babies have never seen their own faces. How do they know what to do to imitate someone sticking out a tongue?" asks Alison Gopnik, professor of psychology at the University of California, Berkeley, and author of *The Philosophical Baby*. We don't know, but they do. "Somehow, the babies are mapping that pink thing sticking outside of someone else, to say here's that thing inside of me."[21]

THE YOUNGEST MIMICS

Newborns are the youngest of mimics. Until the late 1970s, researchers believed that mimicry was a milestone not reached until a baby was about eight months old. Drs. Andrew Meltzoff and M. Keith Moore decided to test infants aged twelve to twenty-one days. Imagine the researchers' surprise when they found that infants just days old could copy facial expressions. When the researchers would stick out their tongues, babies as young as twelve days old would stick out their tongues. The two developmental psychologists, now at the University of Washington in Seattle, showed that even before the babies could see very much, they did their best to replicate the expressions of those studying them. A researcher opened his mouth. So did the baby. A researcher protruded a pouty lip. Baby did, too. It's still not clear how babies know to do this, but they do.

It's that earliest and wordless conversation—the give-and-take of visual communication through imitation of facial gestures—that teaches the baby that what he does gets a response. He's gaining a bit of control over this busy and complicated world that he's entered.

Each time someone smiles at him because he accidentally smiles, or grimaces because he looks pained, or startles because he sneezes, or offers a comforting look because he cries, he's learning that what he does changes the look on the faces of people who care for him. He's learning that he's got the power to communicate. A mother's or father's imitation of him is nothing more than their act of holding up the receiving end of the conversation he's trying to have.

Those marvelous infant eyes, unfocused though they may be, seeing edges through fog, are captivating. They speak loudly to those who love them. Dawn Reeves of Camp Hill, Pennsylvania, the mother of two, recalls eye communication. "I can remember when I felt they were both recognizing my face, even before either one of them truly smiled," she says. "It was the look in their eyes, and I could tell there was recognition there."

It's a difficult and imprecise business, knowing what a baby is seeing or recognizing. But parents and babies have always gazed into one another's eyes. It's deeply rooted, it's bonding, it's complex—and it's important. A look, a simple glance, and we're hooked. They have us way before "hello." They have us at the first opening of the eyes.

CHAPTER SEVEN

Touch

Pain and Pleasure

When my firstborn daughter, Jenny, was three weeks old, she almost died. It was the fall of 1969. I was twenty-one, my husband was twenty-two, and we were living on an army base in Augsburg, West Germany. Jenny had endured a day of projectile vomiting and diarrhea. Her sunken fontanel throbbed, her diaper had been dry for hours, and when I gently pinched her skin it remained wrinkled for several seconds—classic signs of severe dehydration. Beside ourselves with worry, we sped to the emergency room at the base hospital.

The timing for this particular emergency couldn't have been worse. At the time, a few soldiers and their wives were thought to be abusing hospital privileges. Late in a week, they would ask to have their children admitted for ailments like colds or the flu, and then fail to show up for visits until Monday morning. Hospital officials suspected ski weekends in the Alps. So when Jenny became dehydrated, the hospital staff was in the midst of a crackdown. The staff seemed to suspect *everyone* of trying to use the hospital as a babysitting service.

We didn't know all of this when we walked in with Jenny late on a Thursday night. Nurses gave her some water, which this time she managed to keep down—at least as long as the ER visit lasted. The doctor on duty, who seemed annoyed to be awakened, sent us home and told us not to return until the morning, when the clinic opened. For the remainder of the night, Jenny continued to throw up most of what we put in her.

We returned the minute the clinic opened, this time going to the pediatrician's office. He took one look at her, grabbed her from my arms, and shouted, "Follow me," as he ran down the hallway to the pediatric ward.

He recognized the emergency that it was and went right to work, trying to insert a tiny intravenous tube into her veins. When his attempts failed, he ordered us to leave the room. "You won't like hearing her cry, but don't worry. She won't remember the pain."

We left. As we walked down the corridor, I heard a piercing scream from my baby that I will never forget. The doctor performed what he called a cutaway. He made a tiny incision on the inside of her left ankle in order to be able to finally insert the intravenous tube that would deliver lifesaving hydration. In keeping with medical practice of the time, he gave her nothing to ease the pain.

Her father and I were inconsolable as she endured her treatment. Even as I tried to draw solace from the doctor's words, *She won't remember,* the reassurance made no sense. What did he mean? What could memory have to do with that scream that echoed down the hospital corridor and forever in my own memory?

That was more than forty years ago, though it sounds more like a story from the dark ages of medicine. Shocking as it seems, as recently as fifteen years ago, many doctors believed that newborns felt no pain—or in any case, wouldn't remember pain. Nurses lanced their heels, drew their blood, gave them injections, or inserted intravenous tubes. Doctors even performed surgery without any attempt to alleviate pain.

Pain control for newborns has changed dramatically. We now know that the sense of touch is, for forty weeks of pregnancy, influenced by the warmth of amniotic fluid and the secure confines of uterine walls. The transition during the fourth trimester is aided by reminders of those sensations: warm bathing, gentle stroking, swaddling, and cuddling. We can look to sophisticated research showing how infants respond to anesthesia for major procedures and to topical pain-relieving creams for routine care like shots and blood draws. We also know from clinical trials that something as simple and instinctive as holding a baby, skin to skin, can ease discomfort.

BYGONE PAIN THEORY

When I had my babies, doctors had some reason to speculate that newborns didn't feel pain in the same way adults did. Nerve fibers of healthy adults are coated with a substance called myelin. But the immature nerve fibers of infants are not fully coated. Since the myelin coating helps nerves communicate, scientists assumed that newborns were not very good at sending pain signals across nerves. Their brains weren't processing the pain experience in the same way an adult's brain would, they reasoned, and the infant's immature brain wasn't ready to store the memory of the experience.

They were wrong.

We now know that pain pathways from the spinal cord and central nervous system to parts of the brain, including the brain stem and thalamus, are ready to transmit and receive the message of pain by the time a baby is born. While pain signals are carried at a slower pace along the infant's immature nerve fibers, the shorter travel distances in the small body neutralize the slower travel time. Skepticism about infant pain was put to rest in 1987 in a comprehensive review of the medical literature showing that the pathways and chemicals the body uses to feel pain are up and running at birth, and even before birth.[1]

In fact, current research suggests that, rather than feeling less pain in infancy, babies have a higher sensitivity to pain than older children or adults. That's because their bodies' pain-moderating systems are immature. They feel the hurt, but their bodies are not yet equipped to tamp it down. (Those pain-moderating systems seem to be somewhat activated by skin-to-skin contact, though, especially with mothers.)

Medical culture has been slow to change. As recently as 2001, an international group of pediatric and pain experts issued a consensus statement urging pain control when treating infants. "Despite the clinical importance of neonatal pain, current medical practices continue to expose infants to repetitive, acute, or prolonged pain," the statement said. Some health professionals are still unaware of infants' ability to experience pain, or remain fearful of using pain relief measures.[2]

Today, there are guidelines for health professionals to follow, and parents should remind physicians of those guidelines if their infant is going to receive any painful treatment.

PREVENTION AND
MANAGEMENT OF PAIN IN NEWBORNS

1. Pain in newborns is often unrecognized and undertreated. Infants do feel pain, and analgesia should be prescribed when indicated during their medical care.

2. If a procedure is painful in adults, it should be considered painful in newborns, even premature babies.

3. Compared with older age groups, newborns may experience a greater sensitivity to pain and are more susceptible to the long-term effects of painful stimulation.

4. Adequate treatment of pain may be associated with decreased clinical complications and decreased mortality.

5. The appropriate use of environmental, behavioral, and pharmacological interventions can prevent, reduce, or eliminate neonatal pain in many clinical situations.

6. Sedation does not provide pain relief and may mask the neonate's response to pain.

7. Health care professionals have the responsibility for assessment, prevention, and management of pain in neonates.

8. Clinical units providing health care to newborns should develop written guidelines and protocols for the management of neonatal pain.[3]

A BABY CAN FEEL IT

If an adult can feel it, a baby can feel it. We've accepted the belief for years that newborns don't feel pain in the same way that an older child or adult does, but observing an infant in pain contradicts this old myth. Newborns exhibit a set of reactions that we cannot dismiss: cries of distress, flailing, rapid breathing, and elevated heart rate. Most of all, when they feel pain, it's written on their faces. Health professionals now can easily evaluate the distress of babies by consulting a series of photographs showing universal infant reactions to pain.

"The face is the best measure," says Dr. Alyssa Lebel, senior associate in pain medicine at Children's Hospital in Boston. "People have spent an amazing amount of time studying the grimace of the infant."[4]

When infants are in pain, their foreheads crease. Their brows are lowered and drawn close together. Their noses wrinkle. Their eyes squeeze tightly shut. Their mouths open in a square-like shape. Their arms and legs flail. Clinically we can measure the elevation of their heart rates, blood pressure, and breathing rates. Add it together, and it's far different from the cry saying "I'm wet" or "I'm hungry."

Interestingly, most adults can easily identify an infant who is in pain. In one study, about four hundred adults, approximately half of them doctors and nurses and the other half non-health-professionals, were shown photographs of newborns. Some of the pictures were of babies resting; in others, babies were experiencing a light, irritating rubbing; and in others, babies were getting their heels stuck with a needle. The vast majority of adults were able to identify the babies who were feeling pain from the heel stick, though nonprofessionals were better at making the distinction. While 74 percent of doctors and nurses correctly identified the infants in pain, a full 86 percent of nonprofessional adults knew which photos showed infants getting the painful procedure.[5]

The reduced sensitivity shown by health care providers might be a result of their having seen so much pain in their work lives. Studies back up that theory, showing that professionals who routinely carry out painful procedures have a reduced sensitivity to patients' discomfort and become more skeptical of reports of pain. Not so for adults who seldom witness people in pain. Parental instincts usually prove themselves right. Parents and all manner of loving, attentive caregivers know better than anyone when a baby is hurting.

ROUTINE INJECTIONS AND BLOOD DRAWS

Immunizations, blood sampling, and vitamin K injections are routine torments for healthy infants. One study found that newborns who were given just a drop of sugar water on the tongue two minutes before receiving a shot, and who were then held in the arms of a nurse or caretaker during the injection, had significantly less pain, as measured by grimaces and such things as heart rate, than did infants who were held close but didn't get the sugar, or than infants who got the sugar but were not held close.[6]

Sugar is naturally present in breast milk, and breast feeding is as close as anyone can get to a perfect solution for relieving pain from simple procedures. Once again, breast feeding shows itself to be the preferred biological bridge from fetal development to the real world. It combines holding, sucking, skin-to-skin contact, and sugar—all proven ways to reduce infant pain. But formula-feeding parents can provide equivalent comfort by holding the infant, preferably with skin contact, and providing a few drops of sugar water before the baby's ordeal.

The sugar-and-a-hug method costs virtually nothing. While the nurse or doctor is preparing an injection for an infant, there is time to get the infant in a comfortable hold, preferably with some skin-to-skin contact. A breast-feeding mother might begin to nurse. A bottle-feeding parent might have sugar water available in order to place a drop on the baby's tongue or his pacifier. (Never use honey. It can cause botulism in a baby under a year old.)

It's likely that a parent's familiar touch and smell, and the sound of a heartbeat, helps block pain signals from reaching the infant's brain. Or, as shown in animal studies,[7] it may be that the combination of a parent and a bit of sugar fuels the release of an infant's pain-relieving hormones.

CIRCUMCISION

No doubt, the penis is a very sensitive part of the male body. And no doubt, circumcision is a surgical procedure. For the most part, gone are the days when boy babies endured this procedure without regard to their pain.

In 1999, the American Academy of Pediatrics issued a policy statement: "Analgesia is safe and effective in reducing the procedural pain associated with circumcision and, therefore, adequate analgesia should be provided if neonatal circumcision is performed."[8] So don't let a baby go it alone, expecting it to be a character-building experience. It isn't. Talk to a doctor about pain relief. Topical creams like EMLA (a trade name meaning "eutectic mixture of local anesthetics") spread on the penis an hour or so before the procedure can reduce pain. So can a dorsal penile nerve block, which is an injection of lidocaine at the base of the penis. Sugar water on a pacifier or fingertip can help, but this isn't enough in itself to ease the pain of circumcision.

THEY REMEMBER

She won't remember the pain. The sentence lives in my memory, and for decades untold numbers of parents heard it and tried to believe it. "That statement was completely without data," says Dr. Lebel. "It was like a lot of mythology, and it served a purpose. It was comforting [to health care providers] to think that doing things to infants wasn't causing pain."

If it's tactile, good or bad, infants remember. In one study, when newborns in intensive care units who had undergone a lot of needle sticks felt the alcohol swab that was preparing them for yet another stick, they started crying and grimacing before the needle even got close.[9] Already, they knew that a painful stick followed the swab routine. And those who had undergone the greatest number of painful procedures cried harder and grimaced more. Repeated painful experiences resulted in the anticipation of pain, as well as a reduced ability to deal with the pain.

Research conducted over years has shown that people exposed to pain as infants have lower pain thresholds later in childhood. Studies from the 1990s show that infant boys who were circumcised without pain control measures had greater pain responses than uncircumcised boys to routine immunizations performed six months after the circumcision.[10] Rather than the initial pain acting to "man them up," the early experience actually seemed to lower their pain thresholds.

Much of the research on pain and infants has been done in neonatal intensive care units, the subjects being premature or ill infants. But if sick newborns who must endure endless procedures and live with tubes in every orifice of their bodies can suffer less pain through intervention, there's little doubt that there are tools to ease pain in a healthy baby. And on the positive side, there is evidence that infants also remember the soothing, comforting feel of gentle touch.

THE POWER OF TOUCH

The simplest solution is the power of touch. Stroke a baby's cheek, and he'll turn toward the touch. It's one of the first things hospital nurses teach new mothers. Mouth opening and clos- ing, or rooting, may follow, and when a nipple touches the new- born's lips, he'll latch on and suck. It's universal and is part of the Brazelton Neonatal Behavioral Assessment Scale.[11]

Touch his open palm, and he'll grasp your finger. Not only that, his heart rate will slow, indicating that even simple touch has a calming effect. Human-to-human touch is life enhancing, even lifesaving. Studies of premature infants and those exposed to cocaine, as well as of healthy newborns, have found that gen- tle stroking and skin-to-skin touch helps them gain weight and add bone mass faster.

And we do it instinctively and naturally. Almost as though following a guidebook, mothers initially touch their babies in the same way. Orderly and predictable, the physical explora- tion of a newborn infant begins with the mother's fingertips, researchers have observed. Hesitantly, new mothers touch arms and legs, fingers and toes, gently with fingertips. After about four or five minutes, they caress their infants' torsos with the palms of their hands. Gradually, the fingertip touch decreases, and mothers touch, rub, and caress their newborns' entire torsos with their whole hands.[12]

Babies seem to perceive tickling and poking as a sign of peril and generally don't like it. But firm touch and infant massage can reduce crying and distress in newborns. Babies who are massaged tend to sleep longer, and researchers have found they have lower levels of certain stress hormones in their bodies. Massage may also increase another hormone, melatonin, which helps regulate infants' sleeping patterns.[13] A special communication seems to come from touch, with gentle holding and stroking saying, *You are safe,* and poking and jabbing saying, *You're in danger.* For short periods of time, touch can be as profound an attention holder for a newborn as is vision or sound.

There is a neurobiology of pleasure as well as of pain. Remember the initial lack of myelin coating on nerve fibers in newborns? It turns out there are different pathways to unique areas of the brain that carry pleasure signals, and those pathways are less dependent on mature, coated nerve fibers. In adults, hairy skin has fewer of those coated fibers, and scientists have found that stroking hairy skin sends signals to a part of the brain responsible for processing positive emotional feelings. Adults reported more pleasurable feelings when their hairy arms were stroked than when the palms of their hands were stroked.[14] Those studies were done in grown-ups, but it may indicate that the immature nerve fibers in an infant are capable of transmitting soothing, comforting feelings quite well. Think of these alternate signal transmitters as a privileged pathway to pleasure between mothers, fathers, or caretakers and babies. It's a pathway that responds to slow, gentle touch.

As always, watch for a baby's unique response. "He seemed more comfortable with touch on his back. He didn't want as much on his front," says Beth Wheeler of her baby, Matai. "And he didn't seem to like rubbing of his legs." Some babies can't stand to have their heads touched. Others love it. "She loves me touching her face and hair," says Sandy LeBan of her daughter, Natalie. And Molly Lee says of her baby, Abigail: "She doesn't like her feet touched." Maybe, Molly speculates, it's because Abigail spent a few days in the NICU at birth and had an intravenous tube inserted in her foot. For five weeks, her parents changed bandages on the resulting wound, and she may have developed an early aversion to having her feet touched as a result. But Abigail loves gentle massaging strokes on her back and tummy.

So experiment. It won't take long to find out where an infant likes to be touched.

LOVING TOUCH
AND THE DEVELOPING BRAIN

Instinctively, humans sense that touch gives a baby a sense of love, security, and comfort. But it does more than that. It just may trigger activity in her brain that will, shortly down the road, help her to learn better. And farther down that long road of life, early loving touch may provide a child with more resilience against depression and even Alzheimer's disease.

The suggestion of long-term effects such as these comes from a brand-new field called epigenetics, the study of how environmental influence can actually reprogram the expression of genes. (Another hint that the nature/nurture argument has ended in a tie.) While still far from proving that early comforting experiences can help prevent depression and dementia in humans, the new field is beginning to offer intriguing results from animal studies.

In one of the first such studies, researchers from the University of California, Irvine, and Yale University observed thirty-two mother rats and their newborn pups.[15] They recorded the total amount of time mothers spent licking and grooming their infants. Then, in autopsy studies, they examined the baby rats' brains—some in infancy, some late in adulthood. They found that the rats who had been comforted the most, through licking and grooming, had levels of some brain chemicals that were altered in directions associated with decreased stress and increased learning and memory. Those changes lasted into adulthood. The researchers theorize that, in rats anyway, the organization of these stress- and learning- and memory-related neurons may not be hardwired at birth, but rather may be influenced by early experiences.

It turns out that in rats, loving touch can actually modify genes that control a hormone that is a key messenger of stress. The modification can last a lifetime and, as some scientific evidence is beginning to show, may actually be passed on to the next generation.

High stress can increase the release of the corticotropin-releasing hormone, which, in excessive amounts, can lead to a disintegration of some of the brain's connections between neurons. Those connections are responsible for the storage of memories.

As always, it's unwarranted to leap between animal studies and human behavior. But the early findings in rats are no doubt triggering ideas for further research in humans, and the theories and speculation are fascinating. Because a newborn's brain is still building neural connections, large blasts of stress early in life might limit the building of those connections and increase the risk of anxiety, depression, and even dementia later in life. But tender touch reduces the amount of stress-causing hormones in the infant's brain and may give certain types of brain connections—ones that favor memory and learning and protect against stress and depression—a chance to more fully develop.

Every time a baby feels a gentle touch, caress, massage, or nuzzle in a way that pleases the infant, those dendrites that communicate learning and memory are forming and getting stronger, while those that pass on stress signals are getting weaker.

MY FIRSTBORN: EPILOGUE

Jenny still has a tiny scar on her left ankle, and I still carry the scar of guilt. I was young, I had no experience with infants or children, I felt incompetent, and I was overawed by the power of physicians. Back then, I simply would not have questioned the word of a doctor. But I quickly changed. The experience taught me to trust my instincts, even over the orders of an MD. I should have, at the very least, stayed with Jenny and held her in my arms.

As she recovered, she lay in a crib connected to tubes and wires. Neither her father nor I could pick her up, but a caring nurse taught us to lean over the bars of the crib and wrap our arms around her and whisper encouragement. We took turns going home to sleep, and one of us was always there, cradling her, counting the drops that dripped from the intravenous bag into her vein, to be sure the number of drops per minute matched the doctor's orders. She came home strong, to grow and to thrive.

Eighteen years later, when I was unable to talk her out of a tattoo, she chose the image of a rose. She had it placed on the inside of her right ankle. She has no memory of early pain, but I find it fascinating that when she decided to permanently decorate her body with a gentle image, she picked a spot that was the exact counterbalance to the site of her earliest ordeal of pain.

CHAPTER EIGHT

Physical Development

Getting Ready to Crawl, Walk, and Run

Mothers talking:

"Every time she's up, I put her on her stomach for ten minutes to give her a new perspective on the world," says one. "She loves it."

"Sam hates being on his tummy," says another.

"Sometimes mine won't sleep on his back, so I let him fall asleep on his stomach," says a third mother. "Then, when he's sound asleep, I gently turn him over to his back."

"Tummy time," says a fourth, rolling her eyes. "We started from the first month. She wasn't comfortable. It was miserable, and sort of like a comedy. She'd be sprawled out with her face plastered to the floor. I'd crawl down on the floor so she wouldn't be lonely. I don't know what we were accomplishing. I'd rather lay her down on the couch over pillows and play with her that way."

At first, a newborn is not capable of changing his position for his own comfort, much less for his safety. But he struggles mightily. He kicks, he flails, he scrunches and punches—accidental movements that give muscles the serious workout that he needs in order to physically develop. It's important to let an infant practice those muscle-strengthening moves from a variety of positions. In the uterus, he kicked, punched, and even flipped as he grew. The body is growing stronger even as the senses are creating new brain connections. During the fourth trimester, it's up to parents and caregivers to vary their babies' positions in order to let them work those muscles in all directions. After all, during this time of transition infants can't do it by themselves; it's no doubt harder to pull off the moves that might have seemed so easy in the womb.

They're all different, these infants, and it's a challenge to find ways that they enjoy being held. When parents find a position that soothes an infant, who can blame them for wanting to stick to it? But when it comes to positioning—unlike sleeping and eating—the adults in charge can't leave it entirely up to the preferences of newborns. Rather, they have to work to gently convince infants that trying new things will ultimately expand their worlds, even as it strengthens a variety of muscles.

Tummy time is the new addition to the concept "back to sleep," or putting infants down to sleep on their backs. The former in no way negates the importance of the latter, but it's clear that some parents remain confused about how to pull off healthy positioning during the fourth trimester. It's important, during waking hours, to persistently coax an infant into looking at the world from a different angle, into kicking against a surface rather than into the air, and into testing and improving his neck and shoulder strength from a tummy-down position.

The "back to sleep" movement started with a 1994 campaign by the American Academy of Pediatrics, following evidence that prone, or stomach down, sleeping increased the risk of sudden infant death syndrome (SIDS). The campaign increased to 70 percent the number of American babies put down to sleep on their backs. To put it in perspective, a staggering 80 percent of all babies were put down to sleep on their stomachs before the 1994 campaign.[1] But the law of unintended consequences has crept in. Babies who now spend virtually no time in the prone position can experience developmental delays.

THE IMPORTANCE OF "BACK TO SLEEP"

SIDS continues to be one of the major nightmare scenarios for new parents. The cause of the syndrome remains mysterious, but it is abundantly clear that the movement to put babies down to sleep on their backs has dramatically reduced the syndrome's incidence.

The American Academy of Pediatrics first recommended that babies be put down to sleep on their backs in 1992. In 1994, the U.S. government, along with the AAP and several SIDS organizations, launched the "back to sleep" campaign. In 1992, the SIDS rate in the United States was 1.2 deaths per 1,000; by 2002, the rate was .57 per 1,000, or a reduction in SIDS infant deaths of 53 percent.[2]

No one can argue with that kind of success. Positioning isn't the only suspected risk factor for SIDS, however. Sleeping on a soft surface, like a pillow or a feathery mattress, also increases an infant's risk. So does maternal smoking during pregnancy, young maternal age, and a lack of prenatal care, as well as an infant's overheating, low birth weight, and, for unknown reasons, male gender.

So make sure the baby's mattress is firm. She doesn't need a pillow as an infant, nor does she need a crib full of soft, stuffed animals. Those things could put her at risk. Make sure the crib model has not been recalled for safety reasons, and use only the mattress designed for the specific crib, with no gaps between the mattress and the side of the crib. Don't bundle her up too warmly. She shouldn't feel excessively warm during sleep. Suit her up in warm, head-to-toe p.j.'s rather than using blankets.[3]

And put her to sleep on her back.

"BACK TO SLEEP, FRONT TO PLAY"

When babies slept on their stomachs, they got a mild workout of crucial muscles as they moved. To settle themselves, they would lift and turn their heads during the night. This slight movement strengthened the neck, shoulder, and back muscles.

Parents have responded resoundingly well to the advice of physicians to put their infants to sleep on their backs. But some, in their zeal to avoid the nightmare of SIDS, have carried the back message into all hours of the day, including supervised awake time.[4] Pediatric physical therapists and a group called the Pathways Awareness Foundation are concerned about the growing number of babies—an estimated one in forty—being diagnosed with early motor delays.[5] Add to that fear the dazzling array of baby carriers now in use—infant seats, car seats, newborn activity centers, strollers, and swings—and a baby, carried in the parents' arms less often, can end up on his back for most of the first several months of his life.

By 2005, the American Academy of Pediatrics updated its sleep recommendations to take tummy time into account, and tummy time recommendations remain in the newest guidelines, for 2011. These new recommendations continue to stress the importance of putting newborns and infants to sleep on their backs, but they also discuss the importance of supervised tummy time when the baby is awake.

"We have seen firsthand what the lack of tummy time can mean for a baby," says Judy Towne Jennings of the American Physical Therapy Association. "New parents are told of the importance of babies sleeping on their backs to avoid SIDS, but they are not always informed about the importance of tummy time."[6]

But tummy time isn't always well received, especially among very young infants. "For the first month, she wasn't comfortable on her tummy. She didn't even recognize that there were toys around her," says Sandy LeBan. "So I'm staring down at her, wiggling things to get her attention. It was uneventful for her, uneventful for me. My doctor said to do it for five minutes, but for a baby, five minutes is eternity. I could never do it for a full five minutes."

Sandy's solution, to lay Natalie across her lap for tummy time, was perfect. Facedown time doesn't have to be on the floor. It can happen across a parent's lap or in an upside-down arm hold. Whatever works. It doesn't take much—just a few minutes at a time at first.

EVERY MOVEMENT COUNTS

There's a workout going on that no one can see. If parents let their babies spend supervised time on their stomachs early in infancy, then, down the road, they'll sit, crawl, and pull themselves up to stand faster. You can start with just minutes a day for a newborn and work her up to about an hour a day—though not all at one time—on her stomach at three months. One study calculated that if infants spend an hour and twenty-one minutes a day on their stomachs by the age of four months, they'll more quickly reach milestones such as getting up on all fours.[7] But there's no need to get compulsive, no need to set a stopwatch. Instead, encourage tummy time for as long as she enjoys it, several times a day, and figure out ways to incorporate it into her play.

Lying stomach-down puts pressure on a baby's front side. That's obvious, but think about what that is doing. It's forcing him to shift his weight slightly in order to move his head. This slight movement helps him to mobilize the upper spine, and in a few weeks that will help him to lift his head farther and move it to either side.

Prone play and the pressure on the upper trunk also lead to respiratory expansion. In a way, it's exercise for the suck, swallow, and breathing patterns and will someday result in clear speech and articulation. It may not seem like much of an exercise routine, but the slight pressure on the upper trunk caused when an infant lies front-down aids respiratory expansion, which increases lung capacity. That's a benefit in itself, but even as the position is benefiting the lungs, it's also leading to a more mobile rib cage. The benefits of this short and simple daily routine continue to multiply as a more mobile rib cage sets the stage for greater abdominal strength.

Lift up. Hold up. Push up. He's gaining control of his arms and hands. His spine is gaining strength. His hip joints are becoming stable, getting ready to support the entire weight of the body while he stands or walks. It may be hard to believe, but when a baby is on his stomach, he is having a good workout. The simple movements he makes while lying belly-down help the development of his entire upper quadrant, from neck to shoulders to arms. As he gains strength and control during subsequent weeks, he's getting ready for the coordination he'll need to reach for and eventually capture a coveted toy.

During the fourth trimester, parents are most worried about the basics: sleeping, eating, changing, and nurturing. But following just a few simple steps—holding, soothing, and playing with the baby in a variety of positions when she is awake—will benefit future motor development. Start slowly. We're talking minutes, not marathons. Just try to grab a few minutes here and there for this important, alternative position. It won't take long to find positions that please and even amuse the baby.

NO BUCKETS ON THE GROUND

"I look at the devices we build and sell," says Dr. Heidelise Als, director of Neurobehavioral Infant and Child Studies at Children's Hospital in Boston. "That plastic carrying thing is a total depersonalization of the infant. He's strapped into that bucket carrier, and then the same thing goes into the car. He's taken to a babysitter, where the carrier clicks into a stand or a swing device, and the baby never moves. Or they'll put that bucket on the ground. Babies don't belong in a bucket on the ground."[8]

This is not to say that baby containers aren't useful and important—for limited periods of time. They certainly keep baby safe while a parent is driving or when a caretaker has to stir the pot or grab a load of laundry from the dryer. But they are maybe just a bit *too* convenient. Babies can end up spending prolonged periods of time without changing position. One mother told me that her baby slept best in his car seat, so she let him spend many nights there next to her bed. "It was the only way I could get any sleep," she said.

No one could blame her, but I hope it didn't happen too often.

One survey of 187 parents found that 42 percent of infants less than five months old spent between four hours and eight hours of their day in some sort of infant-seating device. Studies have shown that the more time an infant spends in a seating device, the slower she is to reach certain developmental milestones, like rolling over, getting up on all fours, or crawling.[9]

About 15 percent of babies younger than one year receive care in day care centers, and one study showed that infants in day care spend even more time in seating devices than infants cared for at home. In two-hour observations at eight different centers, researchers found that all the babies spent more than half their time in infant seats, swings, or other seating devices. And the younger babies, those five months old and younger, spent up to ninety minutes, or three-quarters of the observed time, strapped into bouncy seats, car seats, or swings, or under stationary activity centers—all on their backs.[10]

LAYING THE GROUNDWORK

So what's the big deal if they crawl later? After all, it means a couple more weeks with fewer concerns about what they're getting into. That may be true, but without ample tummy time, some babies do not crawl at all. Physical development is a sequence of events, one milestone enabling the next.[11] Before they can crawl, they have to strengthen muscles in their necks, their shoulders, their arms, their backs, and their stomachs. It's a chain of physical learning: getting ready to crawl, then stand, then walk, then run.

The chain continues as crawling further strengthens hands, wrists, and shoulders, setting the stage for jungle gym stardom. Crawling also stretches ligaments and develops arches in the hand and wrist. And crawling is experimentation with bilateral coordination, something he'll need forever once he rises onto two feet.

As hard as it may be to imagine as a hapless newborn struggles against gravity while facedown on a lap, he's laying the groundwork in his joints and muscles for the running and jumping that will so delight him later. During the first three months, early positioning for even brief periods of play helps with respiratory expansion, swallowing and breathing patterns, upper body strength, depth perception, and spine and hip strength. It doesn't look like much, those early efforts to raise the head or lift up on the forearms, but it's crucial for all the fun that comes later.

Newborns flail, wiggle, wriggle, thrash, arch their backs, and twitch—all without intention. But accidents help them learn intention. She'll bop a fluffy ball and send it rolling; she'll flail her arms and send an overhead toy swinging, and she'll be overjoyed. It's harder to make these accidents happen while on her tummy, but ultimately she'll get the same glee.

It's the triumph of muscles over gravity. When she starts kicking from a stomach-down position, she's working to stabilize her hip joints. And that's preparing her to someday soon—sooner than a new parent can possibly believe during the demanding days of the fourth trimester—begin to support the entire weight of her body as she pulls herself up on the coffee table. Then, she'll take her first tentative steps. And before you know it, the world is hers to explore.

WORK THOSE MUSCLES

Biceps and elbows, hamstring muscles, toe-lifting muscles, and hip flexors: all those muscles are in a shortened position when infants are in utero. They need stretching. But just as we all are tempted to take the path of least resistance when muscles are tight, a baby will naturally make the movements that are easiest. If his neck muscles encourage him to turn his head to the right, that's what he'll do.

Whatever position an infant is in, an adult can encourage him to look in a different direction. Talk to him from many sides, encouraging him to seek out the familiar voice in various directions. When he's on the changing table, put his head on one side one time, on the other side the next time, so he's using different neck muscles when he turns toward you. And put him down to sleep on his back with his head at one end of the crib one night, the other end the next night. He'll turn toward the light, or toward the sound of a voice, and the different positioning will have him moving a variety of muscles.

He spent nine months in the fetal position, and now he can stretch out those leg muscles. Time spent flat on his stomach gives him a chance to passively do that stretching. The very weight of his body gives those legs a good stretch. At two to three months, as he begins kicking against the floor, he'll be learning the basics of how to push up off a surface. Next thing you know, in an amazing gravity-defying move, he'll try getting up on his elbows, strengthening his shoulder muscles, his core stomach muscles, his abs, and his pecs.

COOL, CALM, PERSISTENT

Eric Kettelhut and his wife, Louisa Elder, learned from Anabelle how much physical therapy she could take and what she refused to tolerate. They followed her cues as she made her way through months of therapy to correct problems with her neck, shoulders, elbows, and hips. Anabelle's physical problems are extreme, and her story is remarkable. But the way Eric and Louisa handled therapy can provide pointers for parents of the healthiest of babies.

The odds were so stacked against Anabelle as she and her twin, Elisa, developed in utero that doctors gave Eric and Louisa no hope that she'd survive until birth. She developed in a sac nearly devoid of amniotic fluid. If she lived to be born, they said, she'd die within minutes or hours. The couple, even as they joyously planned for Elisa's birth, also solemnly made funeral arrangements for Anabelle.

"I believed in my soul that the path for Eric and me was to help welcome one child and help another pass with grace, dignity, and love for both," says Louisa. "This is what I planned for, always hoping against odds that just maybe the baby might survive . . . and she did!" Anabelle astounded everyone. Physicians speculated that the fluid sac around her sister, Elisa, may have cushioned and buffered Anabelle—preventing the uterus from closing around her, as usually happens with inadequate amniotic fluid—giving her just enough space for her lungs to develop.

But she couldn't move. As she developed in the womb, her right arm was contracted. At birth, it would extend forty-five degrees at most. Her neck muscles were so tight she could hardly move her head. She began physical therapy at two days of age. At six months, Anabelle has one arm and her hips in braces.

But she has no neurological problems, smiles as readily as does her sister, and cries as heartily. She's on the mend, all her physical problems fixable—with a lot of daily exercise.

Eric and Louisa have done to an extreme what all parents can do to help their babies' physical development. They have learned how to reposition Anabelle's body in ways that strengthen her muscles—and to do it without making her mad. Or rather, they have learned that when she begins to get upset, it's time to stop, cuddle, comfort, and try something different.

Anabelle had a definite preferred tilt to her neck. When Eric and Louisa first worked with her, they held her head and gently forced it toward the nonpreferred side. Anabelle hated it and cried. So they came up with ideas for strengthening and stretching those shortened neck muscles in ways she didn't mind. They would hold her sideways in their arms, facing front, causing her to lie in a way that gently and passively stretched her head and neck muscles. With every diaper change, they'd position her so that she had to turn her head in the nonpreferred direction to see them.

"Sneakily, we get in those passive stretches," Eric says.

As she got older and developed some strength in her neck, they'd get her comfortable in a sitting position on their laps. When she was happy and content, they'd gently and slightly tip her backward, forcing her chin down. Then, if she was still happy, they'd tip her slightly sideways, strengthening first one side of her neck, then the other. When she cried, they stopped what they were doing. They gave her tummy time, working around her braces and hip cast. By three months of age, she was pushing up on her forearms and lifting her head, moving it side to side.

Anabelle needs a lot more consistent therapy than a healthy baby will. She goes to Pathways Awareness Foundation for physical and occupational therapy five days a week. But the bulk of the effort comes at home, from those subtle holds and cuddling maneuvers that her parents have learned.

Even when physical needs are less extreme, the movement exercises are best done, as Eric says, "sneakily." An exercise can be something as simple as introducing a bottle or pacifier from the side to encourage a neck stretch. If any physical activity makes the baby miserable, stop. Figure out some other way, something that will make it fun for the parent and playtime for baby. Do it naturally, passively—and consistently.

Physical development is an area that may take a bit more conscious attention from parents. Vision develops with normal, everyday exposure to sights, no special toys or equipment required; language develops as a baby hears words and other sounds, including the social interaction of day-in-and-day-out conversation. But physical development depends on someone keeping baby safe by placing her on her back to sleep, and also by giving her time to see the world—and struggle against it— from a tummy-down position.

CHAPTER NINE

Stimulation

Keep It Real, Keep It Simple

Picture a people-pleasing infant wearing a mask of placation and appeasement. Hard as it is to imagine, Dr. Heidelise Als, a neurobehavioral expert at Children's Hospital in Boston, has seen just that in babies as young as three months of age. "Babies who try to please—that breaks my heart," she says. "They have anxious facial expressions. They are good, good—too good, too restricted. They feel performance pressure very early. We see it on videotapes. I see it clinically—the pleasing baby."[1]

Parents will always be somewhat anxious, but the sincere belief that what's needed to stimulate an infant is readily available can tamp down some of that anxiety. Infants don't need to perform in response to flash cards or so-called educational videos. Parents have always found pure enjoyment from hearing their infants freely cooing and gurgling. In fact, videos like the Baby Einstein series, which are aimed at speeding up word acquisition and improving a baby's vocabulary, have been shown to have no vocabulary-improving effect. The younger an infant is when she begins watching the videos, say researchers who studied eighty-eight infants, the lower her language score.[2]

There's no need to buy infant stimulation. Loving attention, comforting touches, eye contact, and closeness to a mother's or caregiver's body—all behaviors that mimic or expand on what the infant experienced in the uterus—provide precisely the stimulation newborns need during the fourth trimester. But society gives new parents ample opportunity to feel confused and guilty.

Companies that make products for babies can exploit common anxiety with seemingly life-altering questions: Are you stimulating your baby enough? Are you providing him with the right tools to develop his mind? Will she be as smart as she can be? Are you blowing his chances of getting into college? Do you have the CDs, videos, toys, mobiles, flash cards, and sound machines that are must-haves if you want your infant to grow up to be smart, happy, and successful?

Relax. During the fourth trimester, everything a baby needs to thrive is available naturally—clouds drifting, rain falling, branches swaying, birds chirping, cats meowing, the morning sun, the shadows of evening. Most important, each baby will thrive in a household—rich, middle-class, or poor—that is filled with love, conversation, affectionate touch, and the smiling faces and responsive attention of parents and caregivers.

DON'T GO OVERBOARD

"We had parents come in with a two-month-old. They brought flash cards with them, cards with dots for counting," says Dr. Russell Hamer, a sensory scientist at the University of São Paulo in Brazil who is also affiliated with the Smith-Kettlewell Eye

Research Institute in San Francisco. In his work, Hamer has seen a steady stream of parents who volunteer to come in with their infants for studies on visual brain waves. "They said they were teaching their baby math. I watched them put their baby through a session. And I'm thinking: 'This baby is only two months old and already has pressure from parents.' I know they're just trying to help accelerate their baby's intellectual development. But something a lot of parents don't understand is that if the environment you generate is unrealistic in a cognitive way, it could have an unwanted negative effect," says Hamer.[3]

At two months, the baby might have seen some grainy dots on a flash card but hardly could be expected to know they were dots, much less how many there were. But the hapless two-month-old is sensitive enough to her parents' expectations to feel their disappointment if she fails to respond to a flash card. A newborn baby has so much to learn. The best way to help her get started is through relaxed and natural interaction.

VISUAL STIMULATION

Evolution has prepared infants to see what they need to see: the shadows of their fathers' eyes, the contrast between an adult's profile and the light behind the head. Infants notice high contrast, like that between the sky and a tree's branches that frame it, or the dark blades of a ceiling fan against the white ceiling. They track the movements of their parents walking across a room. Babies don't need to be distracted, in the name of stimulation, with an abundance of blinking lights or high-contrast toys.

Visual overstimulation is not necessary or beneficial. And for all anyone knows, it might even be harmful—though that, too, is speculation. Again, animal studies offer hints. For example, scientists have shown that visual overstimulation can be bad for baby bobwhite quail and ducklings. In an experiment, hatchlings were exposed to light pulses—levels and patterns of light they would never see in nature. After the exposure, when they were a day and two days old, they failed to recognize their mother's call as normally developing chicks would. It seems that artificial overstimulation of vision interfered with the proper development of another crucial sense: hearing. The chicks were apparently so distracted by the unnatural light that they failed to pay attention to the sound that evolution had equipped them to heed: their mother's peep.[4]

Similar things might happen to a visually overstimulated infant. From birth, infants are better at listening than at looking. They begin to make sense of the world through sounds—words, thumps, and clunks. It's almost as though they need to get a handle on the world one sense at a time.

Dr. Penny Glass, director of the Child Development Program at the Children's National Medical Center in Washington, D.C., says that overstimulation with light, motion, and high-contrast forms can disrupt an important balance between visual learning and auditory learning. Early in her career, her research centered on the effect of bright lights in neonatal intensive care units. The findings, reported in 1985 in the *New England Journal of Medicine*, helped lead to national and international lighting modifications in NICUs. She has since studied environmental effects on all the senses. For babies during the fourth trimester, Dr. Glass advises, "an abundance of brightly colored toys with flashing lights is visually overstimulating. Television is equivalent to staring at multicolored moving lights; videotapes should be avoided entirely, since they provide a stereotyped repetitiveness on multiple viewing not reproducible in nature."[5]

Sure enough, studies have shown that when infants are exposed to high levels of visual stimulation, they are somewhat slower at reaching two milestones: finding their hands and reaching for objects.[6] It may be that it's difficult for infants to disengage their attention from, say, the light of a television screen, and so they don't have the leisure to accidentally notice that they have a hand. Maybe it is something like the neon lights of Las Vegas slot machines distracting a gambler from realizing that someone is picking his pocket.

SOUND STIMULATION

From birth, researchers have found, a newborn recognizes her mother's voice over that of any other woman, this voice no doubt connected to memories made inside the womb. After all, she's heard it in muffled form for nine months. When an infant hears her mother's voice, she will turn in the direction from which it is coming. Just as that familiar face is the most interesting thing in the world for her to see, familiar voices speaking words are exactly what she wants to hear. A parent's voice that she recollects from her time in the uterus, or an adoptive parent's voice that she's come to recognize, will reassure her that someone who loves her is nearby, even if in another room.

If folks in the house like Mozart or classical music or jazz or rock and roll, the newborn is likely to enjoy it, too. But more than music, during the fourth trimester she needs to hear human voices—conversation in the room and, most important, words, coos, and laughs directed to her from loving caregivers.

Human infants learn through social interaction, not from videos, flash cards, or tape recorders. She needs the stimulation of interaction with other people. She'll get it from hearing human voices, and she'll pick up on the give-and-take of conversation as those caring for her respond verbally to her moves, accidental facial expressions, sneezes, and yawns.

TOUCH STIMULATION

Touch is personal. Some babies like having their heads touched but balk at toe touches. Some like their bellies rubbed but not their backs. No special toys or tools are required to stimulate a baby with touch. Make it a relatively firm touch. A light stroke may tickle. Being held, being swaddled, and touching the wooly texture of dad's jacket or the silky softness of mom's blouse all increase the baby's repertoire of sensations.

What a baby needs to grow and develop during the first three months is all right there. Let him feel the chenille on his chest as he notices the contrast of, say, a dark-and-light leaf pattern on a bedspread. Let him touch your face as he looks at you and hears your voice. Help him begin his lifelong exploration of the world by first becoming familiar with the sights, sounds, and textures of the home he has entered.

THE SIX STATES OF AWARENESS

Babies respond in various ways to natural stimulation. How they respond during early infancy depends on differing "states of awareness," as researchers describe them. Learning to recognize those "states" will help caregivers to know what's possible, and what is simply impossible, during certain times. Infants are good at communicating, with varying degrees of subtlety or urgency, which state they are in.

In the 1960s, Dr. Peter Wolff, a child psychiatrist at Harvard Medical School, embarked on a research project with newborns. He spent hours in the homes of infants so he could observe them asleep and awake. Dr. Wolff meticulously recorded their movements and lack of movement. At the same time, Dr. Heinz Prechtl, a developmental neurologist, was conducting a similar study in Holland. Their combined research contributed to the identification of six distinct "states of awareness" among newborns:[7]

Drowsiness

When a newborn is falling asleep—or waking up—he is in a state of drowsiness. He may move, smile, frown, or purse his lips. Before falling asleep, his eyelids appear to be half closed and may roll upward before closing. Give him all the quiet and comfort he needs to start the journey to slumber.

Drowsiness can reappear on awakening, too, when an infant may make some stretching movements. Let him stretch himself out as he begins to get used to the idea of being awake. Adults don't like a lot of insistent demands for socializing when they first open their eyes. Neither does a baby.

Light Sleep

This is also called active sleep, the first stage of sleep for an infant. Her face might be busy with grimaces or sucking motions, and she's easily aroused from sleep. So keep her still and comfortable, and try to keep things as quiet as possible.

Deep Sleep

This is also called quiet sleep. Watch for the calm in her face about half an hour after she falls asleep. The grimaces, accidental smiles, and irregular muscle movements of light sleep calm down. She's deep in slumber.

Quiet Alert

Soon after awakening, a newborn is in a quiet alert state. He may have spent a few seconds in a drowsy state, described earlier, similar to when he was just about to fall asleep. Then his eyes will open wide and bright, but he probably won't move very much. He's putting his energy into seeing and hearing the world around him, so give him a minute to adjust. That's the time to gently hold and rock the baby as he makes the full transition from sleeping to awake.

Active Alert

She'll respond to play, to a voice, to a face. This is the fun time. She might mimic facial expressions or, beginning in the second month, respond to a voice with her own sounds.

But when she's had enough, she'll let everyone know that she's reached her stimulation threshold. She'll squirm, she'll avert her eyes from things that moments before were fascinating, or she'll begin to open and close her hands. She's signaling that, no matter how much mom or dad wants to continue playing, she's ready to stop. Give her a break from play when she seems to be checking out from the stimulation of touch, voice, and face. Put her in a comfortable spot on the floor or a safe and guarded spot on the couch.

Crying

Babies cry. During the first few months of their lives, it is their main way of communicating. Alert caregivers will learn to distinguish between normal crying, crying from distress or pain, and a colicky cry.

The fourth trimester is a time for parents and caregivers to learn their infants' complex and amazingly competent ways of communicating. While paying attention to subtleties, parents will undoubtedly have some episodes of misunderstanding, but everyone—including the newborn—inevitably learns from mistakes.

INDIVIDUAL RESPONSES

Studies of infant development begin with the recognition that all babies are different and respond to stimulation in their own ways. Some are easy and wide eyed; some are excited, eager, and intense; some are sleepy and love quiet time. For all of them, there can be a thin line between the right amount of stimulation and overstimulation. Each baby will react uniquely to being held or swaddled, to the taste of breast milk or formula, the movement of a sister running into the room, the sound of a mother's voice. Every infant has his own capacity and his own limit.

A mellow baby might enjoy a crib mobile. And that may entertain him for a time as he falls asleep. But it may be too much stimulation for an intense baby, who just can't pass up any opportunity to see and hear—rather than sleep. She'll keep herself awake because she can't take her eyes off the fascinating movement of the mobile. Then there are sleepy, quiet-natured babies who may need to be encouraged to pay attention to stimulating sights and sounds. They might need parents to shake a rattle or use their voices to prompt the infant to look around and see.[8]

STIMULATION DEPRIVATION

We have learned a lot from babies deprived of stimulation. In the 1990s, the tragic experiences of orphans in Romania and Russia came to the world's attention and showed neuroscientists how neglect and lack of stimulation can be devastating. These babies spent the first months, even years, of their lives in cribs housed in drab, quiet wards. They wore soiled clothes that didn't fit. Bottles were propped as the infants learned to feed themselves without the comfort of human touch. Their cries, unanswered, changed from signaling need, to signaling desperation and fear, to signaling chronic depression. Eventually, they gave up on crying. Way too many children were under the care of too few adults, and the babies grew up with almost no human touch or stimulation.[9]

Some of those children, later adopted and extensively studied, are still a source of new information on the consequences of early deprivation of stimulation and human connection on physical, behavioral, educational, and social development. When the neglected babies were older, they had poor balance and experienced difficulty coordinating right- and left-side movements. They were, overall, clumsy. They had trouble carrying out instructions involving multiple tasks. Those skills, along with attention and physical dexterity, involve the very areas of the brain—the prefrontal cortex and the cerebellum—that are the last to develop, and which remain undeveloped during the fourth trimester. The extreme treatment of these babies and their complete lack of stimulation affected their development for a lifetime.

THE PERFECT STIMULATION

Normal, everyday life offers the perfect stimulation. Those studies of neglected children provide insights into the need for early stimulation. But babies born into even the poorest of households are at no risk of the kind of understimulation seen in the neglected eastern European orphans. All children, rich or poor, thrive with the stimulation available in natural surroundings. There is virtually no danger of understimulating during the fourth trimester an infant born into a normal household filled with love. All anyone has to do is pay attention to what the baby is trying to say in his primitive, immature, and yet amazingly competent way.

CHAPTER TEN

Mom and Dad

The Parents' Fourth Trimester

From day one, each baby learns how to get his mother's and father's attention. He clings and they hug tighter. He cries, and they say, *Aw, sweetheart, you're okay.* He suckles and his mother relaxes into him. Loving onlookers have counted fingers, toes, and other body parts. They've examined fine hair and miniscule fingernails. Everyone has declared him perfect.

But how are his mother and father doing? How are they *really* doing?

MOTHER'S BODY

When labor begins, the uterus weighs about two pounds, up from two and a half ounces before pregnancy. Immediately after birth, it begins the work of shrinking back down, clamping down, closing off blood vessels in the area where the placenta was attached, and contracting in what feels like cramps. After a week or so, the uterus is down to about a pound in weight, and by four to six weeks it's close to its prepregnancy weight.

If a mother is breast-feeding, it contracts somewhat faster. Her belly is probably still protruding in a kind of pooch because the abdominal muscles have been stretched.

Soon after delivery, the average new mother will be maybe twelve pounds or so lighter. The initial dozen pounds are the easy ones to lose—the weight of the baby herself plus another couple of pounds in blood and amniotic fluid. During the first week after birth, women usually pee a lot, depending on how much water they've retained during pregnancy, and that'll help them drop a few more pounds. But they've no doubt gained additional weight, so they've got some work to do. A reasonable goal is to get back to prepregnancy weight about six months after delivery.

Among women who have delivered vaginally, the vagina will be stretched. Over the next few weeks, it will get smaller, and they can help it along with Kegel exercises. The exercises, named after gynecologist Arnold Kegel, who recommended them back in the 1940s, help tone pelvic-floor muscles, muscles that support the urethra, bladder, uterus, and rectum. Everyone has done these exercises before in life, in order to prevent embarrassment. It's the same kind of muscle squeezing people do when they're trying to stop themselves from passing gas. Combine that squeeze with the one used to stop a flow of urine midstream and *voilà*—the Kegel.

During pregnancy, higher levels of estrogen may have given a woman thicker hair than she's had before. The higher levels of estrogen lengthened the hair's growing phase, and less of it fell out. Now that the baby is here, some of that hair might fall out. In fact, some women shed it in frightening handfuls. Don't worry. The hair's growth and shedding phase will soon return to normal.

Some women have clearer skin during pregnancy, and then break out in acne after the baby is born. Others have uncharacteristic acne during pregnancy, and clear skin after the baby is born. Soon it'll clear up and the skin, too, will be back to normal. Stretch marks, however, are there for the duration. They'll fade in time, but they're one of the lifelong honor badges of motherhood.

Episiotomies are not so common any more, but many women may suffer a tear during delivery. Either way, it takes time to heal. And cesarean sections are increasingly common. Talk to a physician at the postpartum checkup about when to resume sex. Typically couples resume sex after the six-week postpartum checkup, when the first time might make a woman feel like a virgin all over again because of tenderness, dryness, and pain. A water-based lubricant can be a big help.

MOTHERS' BRAINS

Ob-gyns in the past prepared women to expect certain changes in their bodies. But more recently, researchers have used functional magnetic resonance imaging (fMRI) to examine the gray matter of maternal brains shortly after delivery, and they've found that a mother's very brain changes. The changes occur in just those regions—amygdala, thalamus, parietal cortex, and prefrontal cortex—that will help her develop and express the parenting behaviors she'll need for the rest of her life. Those areas support maternal motivation, emotion processing, reasoning, and judgment. Animal studies had earlier shown that the more a mother animal interacts with her offspring, the greater the structural changes in her brain. And now a new fMRI study of human mothers has shown that the same is true for them.[1]

Those who gushed the most, using words like *beautiful, ideal, perfect,* and *special* to describe their infants, and who described their feelings on being mothers as *blessed, content,* and *proud,* experienced greater increases in brain volume in the areas of the midbrain connected with nurturing and sensitivity. The words are universal, as though scripted, but the gushes come from the heart as each mother proclaims her unique welcome.

Researchers speculate that hormonal changes after giving birth—the increases in estrogen, oxytocin, and prolactin—may make the brain more plastic and more susceptible to reshaping itself, actually enlarging areas of the midbrain. Not only do maternal actions help each infant make new and important neural connections, but those very interactions also restructure her own brain, in ways that will help her be a good parent.

CHANGING HORMONES

A woman's body goes through abrupt and dramatic changes in hormonal levels immediately after giving birth. During pregnancy, largely because the placenta is producing estrogens and progesterone, levels of those hormones rise steadily. Two forms of estrogen, estradiol and estriol, increase one-hundred-fold and one-thousand-fold, respectively, during pregnancy. With the removal of the placenta, levels of those hormones drop sharply and suddenly. Levels of other hormones, including beta-endorphin, human chorionic gonadotrophin, and cortisol, also rise to peak levels just before giving birth. They, too, soon plummet when the baby arrives.

In breast-feeding women, levels of prolactin remain at the high levels they reached during pregnancy, and prolactin acts to release oxytocin, a hormone that aids in the contraction of the uterus and stimulates the production of milk. In animal studies, oxytocin has been identified as the body's love-and-cuddle hormone and is linked to maternal nurturing behavior.

The sudden drop in some hormones puts women in an almost menopausal state as far as vaginal dryness is concerned. Most are back to normal in about six weeks, but, as noted earlier, some lubrication might be necessary when they resume sex. Every woman is different, and studies show that women become comfortable with sex anywhere from six weeks to six months after the birth of a baby. But it's the emotional swings caused by sudden changes in hormone levels that are most immediately obvious.

UNBELIEVABLE RELIEF

The extreme emotional reaction of my daughter, Jenny, to giving birth is part of our family lore. I didn't see it but heard about it within an hour of my grandson's birth. In the hospital waiting room, while Jenny was contracting and pushing in the labor and delivery room, I felt like a 1950s sitcom character, pacing, drinking coffee, and waiting for news. Jenny and Chad had tried for seven years to conceive. At last, a few months of acupuncture treatment—or maybe it was an answered prayer or perhaps simply nature's own sweet timing—paid off. They had waited so long for this moment that I knew it should be theirs alone, and after sitting with them through hours of contractions, I left them alone with health care providers to form their new family. Soon after Max's birth, my son-in-law, Chad, invited me into the room, and I held my grandson when he was less than thirty minutes old. Only later did I hear the story of that first half hour.

When Max arrived, Jenny, wan and exhausted, held him. Then a nurse took the baby to a warming table to be cleaned and weighed. Jenny exploded in raw emotion. She laughed out loud and then cried like a banshee. Seconds after a crying jag, and with no apparent transition, she'd start laughing again. Chad said he'd never seen anything like it. He spun back and forth between the warming table, watching his new son, and his wife's bedside, wanting to calm and comfort her. By the time I entered the room, the emotional burst was over. They were all in bed, Jenny holding Max. Chad wrapped the circle of his arm around his wife and baby, both of them studying Max's face while smiling and talking softly.

That moment where laughter and tears were released uncontrollably was no doubt a result of drastic hormonal changes mixing it up with joy and relief. Maybe it had something to do with the nurse taking Max away to the warming table. In any case, it's a story I like to tell Max about how excited his mother and everyone else was the moment he was born.

The moment of birth unfolds differently for every new parent, but no matter how it unfolds, it's a moment that changes everything—forever.

THE BABY BLUES

A baby's entry into the world can be a time when joy coexists with the blues, and that's normal. It's not uncommon to feel mood swings in the days after childbirth. A new mother may feel happy one minute, sad the next. Or she may feel confident one minute, overwhelmed the next. If feelings of sadness or anxiety go away within a few days or a week, it's likely they were the "baby blues."

That's a time to take care. It'll be hard, but new mothers need to find some time to be themselves again. That what Bridget Croke did reluctantly as her husband practically pushed her out the door. "When Alex was two months old, my husband actually kicked me out of the house so I could have some time to myself," says Croke, who lives in Burlington, Vermont. "But when I'm out with friends, I'm constantly checking my cell phone for messages."

Okay, it's fine to check a cell phone. But it's also important to take time to talk to old friends. If they have children, too, then getting together is as important as any business meeting where mothers are doing research and gathering information on how other women are managing things. If friends don't have children, hanging out with them can help a new mother take some time to talk about things other than children.

But if a woman feels depressed, worthless, restless, anxious, and fatigued for longer than a couple of weeks, it may interfere with her ability to care for or bond with her baby. That's when it's time to seek out additional help.

EARLY CLUES
OF POSTPARTUM DEPRESSION RISK

Postpartum depression is common. According to the Centers for Disease Control and Prevention, one in ten women is depressed during any trimester of pregnancy or any month during the first year after delivery.[2] In a study of about forty-four hundred women, the CDC found that more than half of the women who suffered postpartum depression had been depressed during pregnancy or shortly before they got pregnant. Another federal agency, the Agency for Healthcare Research and

Quality, found that 15 percent of mothers are depressed during the first three months after giving birth.[3] Finding and treating depression early can help both mother and baby get on with the important work of bonding and falling in love.

The most common method of diagnosis is the Edinburgh Postnatal Depression Scale, a standardized scale that consists of ten questions zeroing in on feelings over the previous ten days. When physicians use a formal screening tool such as this, it increases the odds of accurately diagnosing and treating depression. The questions assess a woman's ability to laugh and enjoy, as well as her level of worry, fear, or sadness or of being overwhelmed. Scoring the answers helps physicians determine if their patients are depressed.

Family physicians or pediatricians can screen a mother at her baby's first well-baby visit, at about two weeks of age, but studies show that fewer than half of physicians do such screening.[4] It can also be done at the first postpartum exam at about six weeks after the birth—a bit late for a woman who may be suffering from postpartum depression. And even if a woman's test result indicates she's depressed, physicians often fail to follow up or give her a mental health referral.

TREATING POSTPARTUM DEPRESSION

Psychotherapy, support, and talk work for many; for some, drugs can help. Some states require postpartum depression screening, and the new health reform law has provisions for additional research, patient education, and support for mothers who have depression. But it still may be up to the individual woman to seek help. A woman should pay attention if a partner, or close family members, or friends tell her that they sense something is amiss in her response to her baby. Symptoms include loss of appetite, insomnia (inability to sleep even when baby is sleeping), irritability, anger, severe fatigue, lack of joy, feelings of shame or guilt, withdrawal from family and friends, and an inability to bond with the baby.

Treatment may come in the form of a support group or psychotherapy. The Cochrane Collaboration is an international network of experts providing systematic reviews of primary research papers in health care and health policy. In its recent review of nine studies involving more than nine hundred women, a Cochrane review found that peer support such as mothers' groups and psychotherapy reduced symptoms of depression.[5] Antidepressant drugs can be used, says Mary Kenny, a nurse and social worker who works with postpartum patients at Loyola University Medical Center, but only under a physician's, preferably a psychiatrist's, close care. "There are some women who just can't function without being on meds," says Dr. Aparna Sharma, a psychiatrist with Loyola who works with women who have postpartum depression.[6] Each woman, with her physician, must then make a decision, balancing the need for antidepressant medication with the baby's needs. The drugs make their way into breast milk, so many women will have to decide not to breast-feed if they need medication, or to postpone medication because they want to breast-feed.

ON THE RESEARCH HORIZON

There are other measures that might soon help find women at high risk for postpartum depression before it ever hits.

Almost every woman remembers that first ultrasound, the first time she saw the fetus inside make a fist or wiggle a toe.

Those early photographs of fetuses are now a common early gateway to parenthood. They show up framed on desktops, held with magnets on refrigerators, or pasted as the first entry in a baby book. Studies have shown that those early glimpses increase attachment and promote early bonding. They can be a deciding factor in convincing women to quit smoking and avoid drinking alcohol.

Unfortunately, ultrasounds are also used politically, when it comes to women who have made a difficult decision to terminate a pregnancy. Despite no medical evidence supporting the need for an ultrasound before a first-trimester abortion, twenty states regulate the provision of ultrasound services by abortion providers and eleven more states require that verbal counseling or written materials include information on accessing ultrasound services as part of preabortion counseling. Some women who know they are not ready, equipped, able, or willing to become mothers may feel coerced into undergoing a medically unnecessary procedure, presumably intended to impose a bonding process.[7]

But many women are ready for that first peek inside the uterus. Alexandria Stockman, a graduate student working on a PhD in clinical psychology at the Illinois Institute of Technology, watched more than two hundred women as they saw their fetuses for the first time during ultrasound screenings.[8] Women talked to the screens. Sometimes they reached out and touched the screens. Stockman was in the room and so were two cameras, one focusing on the screen, the other on the mother. Stockman took notes.

"Me and baby, we don't miss a meal," laughed one. "He's kicking. When he kicks, he's telling me he's hungry." She rubbed her tummy as she looked at the screen.[9]

"Wow, she just grabbed her toe."

"Oh, I always wanted a girl." Or: "Oh boy, it's a boy."

"That's my nose. She has my nose."

"Look, he's flipping over. He's going to be an athlete."

These snippets of conversation represent the first multi-level interaction going on via technology. "Look at you, Jason. I can't believe you're so agile in there." When women are able to interact with the fetus that early in pregnancy, Stockman speculates, it's a good sign that they're ready for motherhood.

But some women look away from the image. They don't talk to or about the fetus they're seeing on the screen. Those women are showing early signs of not being prepared for motherhood. They may be in the midst of processing a difficult and highly personal decision to either proceed with or terminate the pregnancy. If they proceed with the pregnancy, they may have increased trouble bonding with the baby when he's born, or they may be more likely to suffer from postpartum depression.

Stockman works with researcher Dr. Zachariah Boukydis of the Erikson Institute in Chicago. They found that women with higher levels of anxiety and depression early in their pregnancies were less interested in the image on the screen. They also were more likely to say negative things about the fetus: "I don't like the position he's in" or "She kicked me so hard I almost fell over." These are women who might benefit from counseling early on. It's possible that some women could be spared postpartum depression or could confront their doubts about motherhood before the baby is born. "The response to the ultrasound gives you a picture of how the woman is holding the baby in her mind," says Stockman.

A blasé or negative response to an ultrasound image may be one clue that a woman is especially vulnerable to postpartum depression. Research has shown early indications of a second clue. About halfway through pregnancy, the placenta produces a hormone called placental corticotropin-releasing hormone, or pCRH. In a study of one hundred pregnant women, blood samples were taken at various stages of pregnancy.[10] It turned out that at twenty-five weeks' gestation, if a woman's level of this hormone was unusually high, there was a good chance she'd go on to suffer postpartum depression. Screening women's pCRH levels is not now part of prenatal care; but if the research findings are replicated, it's possible that this screening could take place at the same time that blood screening is done for gestational diabetes—at about twenty-four to twenty-eight weeks.

NIGHTMARES, FEARS, AND OBSESSIVE CHECKING

Even more common is perinatal anxiety, and it hits fathers as well as mothers. It stands to reason that such anxiety could touch adoptive parents as well as biological parents. I still remember a vivid dream I had shortly after my first child was born. I dreamed that I looked into her cradle and saw a tiny foot growing from the middle of her nose. It was horrifying, the kind of nightmare that makes you wake up in a sweat, heart pounding. A lot of new mothers and fathers have dreams, nightmares, or daytime anxiety that keeps them on pins and needles with worry. Is something wrong with my baby? Am I a good enough parent? Perinatal anxiety is less discussed, but perhaps more common, than postpartum depression.

Most people can dismiss such thoughts or dreams and move on. But if these interfere with sleep or with the ability to care for the baby, talk to a doctor and get help.

DADS GET
POSTPARTUM DEPRESSION, TOO

Mood downturns among fathers are far less studied than postpartum depression in mothers, but it's becoming clear that this problem exists. Dr. James F. Paulson and Annie Panno of the Eastern Virginia Medical School in Norfolk, Virginia, examined forty-three studies involving more than twenty-eight thousand fathers.[11] Their findings showed that about 10 percent of fathers experience depression between the mothers' first trimester of pregnancy and the first year after a child was born. That's more than double the average depression rate for adult men, which is 4.8 percent. Rates were highest among fathers when the baby was between three and six months old. When the mother was depressed, this increased the chance that the father too would experience depression.

New fathers—or any adult responsible for the twenty-four-hour care of a newborn—are sleep deprived, too, and that alone can alter neurochemical balances in the brain, making anyone more vulnerable to an episode of depression. If a new mother is feeling blue, her spouse would do well to check his own emotional response. Even if a woman is showing no signs of depression, a new father might look for the signs in himself: loss of appetite, insomnia, irritability, anger, severe fatigue, lack of joy, feelings of shame or guilt, withdrawal from family and friends, or an inability to bond with the baby. Some mental health experts suggest screening for postpartum depression in both parents, not just mothers.

THE IMPACT
OF FATHERHOOD ON MEN'S HEALTH

Men's health is a relatively new field of study, and the specific health impact of fatherhood on men is an area that is all but untouched. We do know that men often report feeling unprepared for fatherhood. An Australian study of 312 men, called the First-Time Fathers Study, found that their spouses' pregnancies were more stressful than the births of the children. The study also found a significant deterioration in sexual activity during pregnancy and the first year of the child's life.[12]

A September 2004 review of medical studies, published in the *Journal of Men's Health and Gender,* found a variety of trouble spots for men during pregnancy, labor and delivery, and the first year of fatherhood.[13] It's uncommon but not rare, for example, for some men to experience some of the same symptoms their wives are feeling during pregnancy, like nausea or constipation. During labor and delivery, a significant number of men report feeling ill-prepared, ineffective, or disregarded. And when baby comes home, most men experience an emotional upheaval as they adapt to the presence of a family member who needs full-time attention and care.

But the good news is that fatherhood, over the long haul, is beneficial to a man's health.

FATHERHOOD: HUMOR CAN'T HURT

Dads get overlooked. They may be even more awkward than moms when holding, comforting, and diapering a newborn. A dad may do things differently. Let him. Maybe a different kind of hold, a varied firmness, will soothe the baby. It will teach the baby that there's more than one person who loves him, and it will show the baby that there is more than one right way to do things.

A quick overview of books to help men prepare for fatherhood shows little of the gravitas afforded new mothers. Many of the titles make tongue-in-cheek references to fear, panic, or basic survival: *Dada: A Guy's Guide to Surviving Pregnancy, Childbirth and the First Year of Fatherhood,* by Michael Crider; *She's Having a Baby—and I'm Having a Breakdown,* by James D. Barron; *The New Father's Panic Book: Everything a Dad Needs to Know to Welcome His Bundle of Joy,* by Gene B. Williams; *Keeping the Baby Alive till Your Wife Gets Home: The Tough New 'How-To' for 21st Century Dads,* by Walter Roark.

When a young friend, and first-time father, received such an advice book, this conversation followed: "Thanks, man, I need this," said the new father. "Yeah, it helped me a lot," responded the young man who'd recently been there. They may be men of few words, but they were savvy enough to help each other out.

THE STRAIN ON COUPLES

I don't want to rain on any new parent's parade, but I do want couples to be realistically prepared. So here it is: parenthood hastens marital decline. That depressing finding flies in the face of greeting card images and advertisements depicting robust babies and their adoring, smiling parents. But new parents can understand that when everything changes, some of the changes are not good. They get less sleep. They spend less intimate time with their mate. They have less time, maybe no time at all, to do the things they've always loved doing: biking, playing golf, and going to movies, concerts, or plays. Knowing the extent of the challenge to couples is important if mothers and fathers are to successfully navigate the fourth trimester and beyond.

As early as 1957, E.E. LeMasters, a researcher from Beloit College, in Beloit, Wisconsin, showed that 83 percent of new parents experienced a moderate to severe crisis soon after the birth of a baby.[14] Later studies have found that, while the arrival of children can also bring joy and pleasure, even couples in the healthiest of relationships can shift roles, change focus, and undergo stress. For almost all mothers and fathers, it's a desired and welcome change that nonetheless isn't easy.

A lot of research has been done on the effect of children on relationships, asking couples to rate their happiness and satisfaction after they had children and then again as the children got older. In a 2008 study aimed at comparing the relative happiness of couples who have children with that of childless couples, researchers from the University of Iowa recruited 104 couples and followed them from some point within the first six months of their marriage through the twelve months after the birth of their first child. For comparison, they also recruited 52 couples who did not want to have children and followed them from the first six months of marriage through the next four years. All couples were given questionnaires on marital satisfaction and were rated at various and similar points in time on a standard measure called the Quality of Marriage Index.[15]

All participants, whether parents or childless couples, reported less marital satisfaction at the end of the four-year study than they did in the first six months of marriage. That's probably not surprising. Honeymoons do end. But the satisfaction slide was steeper for fathers and mothers than it was for husbands and wives who didn't have children. On a scale of satisfaction that runs from a low of 6 (pretty miserable) to 45 (ecstatic), marital satisfaction declined within the studied time frame by 2.73 points for nonparent husbands, but by 5.07 points for husbands who were fathers; marital satisfaction for nonparent wives slid by 2.34 points but fell further—5.07 points—when the wives were mothers. When the pregnancy was unplanned, the decline in marital satisfaction was greater, especially for fathers.

Other studies have found that marital dissatisfaction peaks when the child is a year old, and slowly begins to rebound during the child's second year.

These findings aren't meant to frighten couples, but rather to prepare them for a transition that could well be bumpy. And take heart. An infant's arrival is as unlikely to destroy a first-rate marriage as it is to miraculously fix a troubled relationship.

REINFORCEMENTS WELCOME

Husbands and wives may have worked hard to become a team in their marriage, formulating and working toward common goals. Each one tries new things for the sole reason that the other likes them—tennis, Brussels sprouts, mystery fiction, or noir movies. After all, sharing interests increases the opportunities to do things together.

Now, the baby is here and there are fewer opportunities to team up as a couple enjoying things together. Everyone has a big job ahead, and it's going to take the coordinated effort of both partners, whether married or not, gay or straight. A couple is still a team, but as one young mother told me, maybe for a while they're more of a tag team. Mom runs to the supermarket while dad walks the floor with the infant. She comes home, and rocks and feeds the baby while dad stuffs in a load of laundry. Perhaps most crucial, one partner sleeps while the other takes a shift with the baby, then she wakes up and takes the torch of responsibility while dad gets some sleep.

Now that team needs reinforcement. This is no time for go-it-alone isolation. Lean on health care providers for medical assurance; for all else lean on family, friends, neighbors, baby-sitters, nannies, and grandparents—anyone who can be counted on to love the new family. As our society's definition of *family* changes from simply "husband, wife, and children" to one that includes single parents, gay parents, separated and divorced parents, combined families, and stepfamilies, love from any quarter can only serve to enhance a baby's experience.

Science will continue to strive to lift the cloak of mystery surrounding the inner workings of newborn humans, and knowledge will only enhance the awesome experience of caring for a brand-new baby.

It's transformative. There is nothing else like it.

NOTES

INTRODUCTION

1. Throughout the book, I quote parents from my interviews with them, which were recorded in 2009 and 2010, unless otherwise noted.

2. National Research Council and Institute of Medicine Committee on Integrating the Science of Early Childhood Development, Jack P. Shonkoff and Deborah A. Phillips, eds., Board on Children, Youth, and Families, Commission on Behavioral and Social Sciences and Education, *From Neurons to Neighborhoods: The Science of Early Childhood Development* (Washington, DC: National Academy Press, 2000).

3. Wenda R. Trevathan and James McKenna, "Evolutionary Environments of Human Birth and Infancy: Insights to Apply to Contemporary Life," *Children's Environments* 11, no. 2 (June 1994): 13–36.

4. James J. McKenna, *Sleeping with Your Baby: A Parent's Guide to Cosleeping* (Washington, DC: Platypus Media, 2007).

5. Joseph McVicker Hunt, *Intelligence and Experience* (New York: Ronald Press, 1961).

I. EVOLUTION AND
THE PRIMITIVE BRAIN OF A NEWBORN

1. Ker Than, "'Lucy's Kin Pushes Back Evolution of Upright Walking?" *National Geographic News,* June 21, 2010.

2. Dr. Wenda Trevathan, interview by author, December 21, 2009. All quotes by Dr. Trevathan in this chapter are from this interview.

3. Ashley Montagu, *Touching: The Human Significance of the Skin* (New York: HarperCollins, 1986). Anthropologist Dr. Ashley Montagu, who coined the term *exterogestation,* to contrast with *uterogestation,* the nine months with which we're all familiar, was notable for shifting traditional thinking toward the idea of a fourth trimester of outside-the-womb development.

4. Karen R. Rosenberg and Wenda R. Trevathan, "The Evolution of Human Birth," *Scientific American* (November 2001): 77–81.

5. National Institutes of Health, "The Life and Death of a Neuron," n.d., www.ninds.nih.gov/disorders/brain_basics/ninds_neuron.htm, accessed May 7, 2012.

6. P.R. Huttenlocher, "Synaptic Density in Human Frontal Cortex—Developmental Changes and Effects of Aging," *Brain Research* 163 (March 16, 1979): 195–205; and P.R. Huttenlocher and A.S. Dabholkar, "Regional Differences in Synaptogenesis in Human Cerebralcortex," *Journal of Comparative Neurology* 387 (October 20, 1997): 167–178.

7. Nathan A. Fox, Lewis A. Leavitt, and John G. Warhol, eds., *The Role of Early Experience in Infant Development,* Johnson and Johnson Pediatric Institute Pediatric Round Table Series, 1999, www.baby.com/jjpi/for-professionals/The-Role-of-Early-Experience-in-Infant-Development.pdf, accessed May 7, 2102.

8. National Institutes of Health, "The Life and Death of a Neuron."

9. Joe L. Frost, "Neuroscience, Play, and Child Development" (prepared for presentation at the International Play Association USA Triennial National Conference, Longmont, Colorado, June 18–21, 1998).

10. National Institutes of Health, "The Life and Death of a Neuron."

11. National Research Council and Institute of Medicine Committee on Integrating the Science of Early Childhood Development, Jack

P. Shonkoff and Deborah A. Phillips, eds., Board on Children, Youth, and Families, Commission on Behavioral and Social Sciences and Education, *From Neurons to Neighborhoods: The Science of Early Childhood Development* (Washington, DC: National Academy Press, 2000), 186.

12. Natalie Angier, "The Purpose of Playful Frolics: Training for Adulthood," *New York Times,* October 20, 1992.

13. Dr. James McKenna, interview by author, October 5, 2009.

14. John Bowlby, *Attachment and Loss,* vol. 1 (New York: Basic Books, 1969).

2. CRYING

1. Anne Lamott, *Operating Instructions: A Journal of My Son's First Year* (New York: Anchor Books, 1993), 36.

2. Jerome Groopman, "The Colic Conundrum," *New Yorker,* September 17, 2007.

3. Barry Lester, *Why Is My Baby Crying?* (New York: Harper-Resource, 2005).

4. J. Bowlby, *Attachment and Loss,* vol. 1 (New York: Basic Books, 1969).

5. Konrad Lorenz, *Studies in Animal and Human Behavior* (Cambridge, MA: Harvard University Press, 1971).

6. Melanie L. Glocker, Daniel D. Langleben, Kosha Ruparel, James W. Loughead, Jeffrey N. Valdez, Mark D. Driffin, Norbert Sachser, and Ruben C. Gur, "Baby Schema Modulates the Brain Reward System in Nulliparous Women," *Proceedings of the National Academy of Science* 106 (April 2009): 9115–9119.

7. Dr. Heidelise Als, interview by author, December 7, 2009.

8. Heidelise Als, "The Newborn Communicates," *Journal of Communication* 27 (Spring 1977): 66–73. For an interview explaining her early studies of those interactions, see www.brazelton-institute.com/abinitio2009spring/art3.html.

9. Maureen R. Keefe, Kristine A. Kajrlsen, William N. Didley, Marie L. Lobo, and Anne Marie Kotzer, "Reducing Parenting Stress in Families with Irritable Infants," *Nursing Research* 55, no. 3 (May–June 2006): 198–205.

10. Lester, *Why Is My Baby Crying?* A colic researcher, Dr. Lester draws on his experience as the founder of the Colic Clinic in Providence, Rhode Island, to offer science-based information.

11. Harvey Karp, *The Happiest Baby on the Block* (New York: Bantam, 2002). This best-selling book introduced the concept of the five S's to soothe a crying child.

12. Dr. Linda Gilkerson, interview by author, October 19, 2009.

13. Michelle Lee Murrah, interview by author, March 9, 2010. All quotes by Murrah in this chapter are from this interview.

14. Dr. Heidelise Als, interview by author, December 7, 2009.

15. E.M. Baildam, V.F. Willer, B.S. Ward, R.P. Bannister, F.N. Bamford, and W.M.O. Moore, "Duration and Pattern of Crying in the First Year of Life," *Developmental Medicine and Child Neurology* 37 (April 1995): 345–353.

16. Ann M. Frodi, Michael E. Lamb, and Diane Wille, "Mothers' Responses to the Cries of Normal and Premature Infants as a Function of the Birth Status of Their Own Child," *Journal of Research in Personality* 15, no. 1 (March 1981): 122–133.

3. SLEEPING

1. Dr. James McKenna, interview by author, October 17, 2010. All quotes by Dr. McKenna in this chapter are from the same interview.

2. Carolyn C. Thiedke, "Sleep Disorders and Sleep Problems in Childhood," *American Family Physician* 63, no. 2 (January 15, 2001): 277–285.

3. Ivo Iglowstein, Oskar G. Jenni, Luciano Molinari, and Remo Largo, "Sleep Duration from Infancy to Adolescence: Reference Values and Generational Trends," *Pediatrics* 111, no. 2 (February 2003): 302–307.

4. Rodrigo Jose Custodio, Carlos Eduardo Martinelli Junior, Soraya Lopes Sader Milani, Aguinaldo Luis Simoes, Margaret de Castro, and Ayrton Custodio Moreira, "The Emergence of the Cortisol Circadian Rhythm in Monozygotic and Dizygotic Twin Infants: The Twin Pair Synchrony," *Clinical Endocrinology* 66, no. 2 (February 1, 2007): 192197.

5. Linda C. Mayes and Donald J. Cohen, *The Yale Child Study Center Guide to Understanding Your Child* (New Haven, CT: Yale University Press, 2002), 170.

6. Thomas F. Anders, "Organization and Development of Sleep in Early Life," *Encyclopedia on Early Childhood Development,* published online January 12, 2004; rev. March 19, 2010, accessed May 8, 2012.

7. Harvey Karp, *The Happiest Baby on the Block* (New York: Bantam, 2002).

8. Barak E. Morgan, Alan R. Horn, and Nils J. Bergman, "Should Neonates Sleep Alone?" *Biological Psychiatry* 70 (November 2011): 817–825.

9. James J. McKenna and Thomas McDade, "Why Babies Should Never Sleep Alone: A Review of the Co-sleeping Controversy in Relation to SIDS, Bedsharing and Breast Feeding," *Paediatric Respiratory Reviews* 6 (2005): 134–152.

10. James J. McKenna et al., "Sleep and Arousal Patterns of Co-sleeping Human Mother-Infant Pairs: A Preliminary Physiological Study with Implications for the Study of Sudden Infant Death Syndrome (SIDS)," *American Journal of Physical Anthropology* 83 (March 1990): 331–347.

11. Lee T. Gettler and James J. McKenna, "Never Sleep with Baby? Or Keep Me Close But Keep Me Safe: Eliminating Inappropriate 'Safe Infant Sleep' Rhetoric in the United States," *Current Pediatric Reviews* 6, no. 1 (February 3, 2010): 71–77.

12. Kristine McCulloch, Robert T. Brouilette, Anthony J. Guzzetta, and Carl E. Hunt, "Arousal Responses in Near-Miss Sudden Infant Death Syndrome and in Normal Infants," *Journal of Pediatrics* 101, no. 6 (December 1982): 911–917.

13. M.M. Vennemann, T. Bajanowski, B. Brinkmann, G. Jorch, K. Yucesan, C. Sauerland, E.A. Mitchell, and the GeSID Study Group, "Does Breastfeeding Reduce the Risk of Sudden Infant Death Syndrome?" *Pediatrics* 123, no. 3 (March 1, 2009): e406–e410.

14. James McKenna, *Sleeping with Your Baby: A Parent's Guide to Co-sleeping* (Washington, DC: Platypus Media, 2007).

15. James J. McKenna, Helen L. Ball, and Lee T. Gettler, "Mother-Infant Cosleeping, Breastfeeding and Sudden Infant Death Syndrome:

What Biological Anthropology Has Discovered about Normal Infant Sleep and Pediatric Sleep Medicine," *Yearbook of Physical Anthropology* 50 (2007): 133–161.

16. James J. McKenna, "Cultural Influences on Infant and Child-hood Sleep Biology and the Science That Studies It: Toward a More Inclusive Paradigm," in *Sleep in Development and Pediatrics*, ed. J. Loughlin et al. (New York: Marcel Dekker, 1999).

17. William Sears and Martha Sears, "SIDS: The Latest Research on How Sleeping with Your Baby Is Safe," Ask Dr. Sears, www.askdrsears.com/topics/sleep-problems/sids-latest-research-how-sleeping-your-baby-safe, accessed May 8, 2012.

18. For the American Academy of Pediatrics' recommendation, see Task Force on Sudden Infant Death Syndrome, "The Changing Concept of Sudden Infant Death Syndrome: Diagnostic Coding Shifts, Controversies Regarding the Sleeping Environment, and New Variables to Consider in Reducing Risk," *Pediatrics* 116, no. 5 (November 2005): 1245–1255.

19. American Academy of Pediatrics, Task Force on Sudden Infant Death Syndrome, "SIDS and Other Sleep-Related Infant Deaths: Expansion of Recommendations for a Safe Infant Sleeping Environment," *Pediatrics* 128, no. 5 (November 1, 2011): e1341–e1367.

20. McKenna, *Sleeping with Your Baby*, 61–69 .

4. FEEDING

1. M. M. Vennemann, T. Bajanowski, B. Brinkmann, G. Jorch, K. Yucesan, C. Sauerland, E. A. Mitchell, and the GeSID Study Group, "Does Breastfeeding Reduce the Risk of Sudden Infant Death Syndrome?" *Pediatrics* 123, no. 3 (March 1, 2009): e406–e410.

2. Stanley Ip, Mei Chung, Gowri Raman, Priscilla Chew, Nombulelo Magula, Deirdre DeVine, Thomas Trikalinos, and Joseph Lau, *Breastfeeding and Maternal and Infant Health Outcomes in Developed Countries*, Evidence Report/Technology Assessment No. 153, AHRQ Publication No. 07-E007 (Rockville, MD: Agency for Healthcare Research and Quality, April 2007), accessed May 8, 2012.

3. Mary L. Hediger, Mary D. Overpeck, Robert J. Kuczmarski, and W. June Ruan, "Association between Infant Breastfeeding and Overweight in Young Children," *Journal of the American Medical Association* 285, no. 19 (May 16, 2001): 2453–2460.

4. Michael S. Kramer, Beverley Chalmers, Ellen D. Hodnett, Zinalda Sevkovskaya, Irina Dzikovich, Stanley Shapiro, Jean-Paul Collet, Irina Vanilovick, Irina Mezen, Thierry Ducruet, George Shishko, Vyacheslav Zubovich, Dimitri Mknuik, Elena Gluchanina, Viktor Dombrovskly, Anatoly Ustinovitch, Tamara Kot, Natalia Bogdanovich, Lydia Ovchinikova, and Elisabet Helsing, "Promotion of Breastfeeding Intervention Trial (PROBIT): A Randomized Trial in the Republic of Belarus," *Journal of the American Medical Association* 285, no. 4 (January 24–31, 2001): 413–420.

5. Michael S. Kramer, Frances Aboud, Elena Mironova, Irina Vanilovich, Robert W. Platt, Lidia Matush, Sergei Igumnov, Eric Fombonne, Natalia Bogdanovich, Thierry Cucruet, Jean-Paul Collet, Beverley Chalmers, Ellen Hodnett, Sergei Davidovsky, Oleg Skugarevsky, Oleg Trofimovich, Ludmila Kozlova, and Stanley Shapiro for the Promotion of Breastfeeding Trial (PROBIT) Study Group, "Breastfeeding and Child Cognitive Development," *Archives of General Psychiatry* 65, no. 5 (May 2008): 578–584.

6. Siobhan Reilly and Eirik Evenhouse, "Improved Estimates of the Benefits of Breastfeeding Using Sibling Comparisons to Reduce Selection Bias," *Health Services Research* 40 (December 2005): 1781–1802.

7. M. Ines Klein, Eduardo Bergel, Luz Gibbons, Silvina Coviello, Gabriela Bauer, Alicia Benitez, M. Elina Serra, M. Florencia Delgado, Guillermina A. Melendi, Susana Rodriguez, Steven R. Kleeberger, and Fernando P. Polack, "Differential Gender Response to Respiratory Infections and to the Protective Effect of Breast Milk in Preterm Infants," *Pediatrics* 121, no. 6 (June 1, 2008): e1510–e1516.

8. Ip, Chung, Raman, Chew, Magula, DeVine, Trikalinos, and Lau, *Breastfeeding and Maternal and Infant Health Outcomes in Developed Countries.*

9. Adriano Cattaneo, "The Benefits of Breastfeeding or the Harm of Formula Feeding?" *Journal of Pediatrics and Child Health* 44 (January–February 2008): 1–2.

10. Dr. James McKenna, interview by author, October 5 and 17, 2009.

11. Prashant Gangal, "Initiation of Breastfeeding by Breast Crawl," n.d. Video available at http://breastcrawl.org/contributors.shtml, accessed May 8, 2012.

12. Wen-Jui Han, Christopher J. Ruhm, Jane Waldfogel, and Elizabeth Washbrook, "The Timing of Mothers' Employment after Childbirth," *Monthly Labor Review* 131 (June 2008): 15–26.

13. American Academy of Pediatrics, "Policy Statement: Breast-feeding and the Use of Human Milk," *Pediatrics* 115, no. 2 (February 1, 2005): 496–506.

14. Centers for Disease Control and Prevention, "Breastfeeding Report Card 2011, United States: Outcomes Indicators," August 1, 2011, www.cdc.gov/breastfeeding/data/reportcard2.htm, accessed May 8, 2012.

15. Jody Heymann, Alison Earle, and Jeffrey Hayes, *The Work, Family, and Equity Index: How Does the United States Measure Up?* (Montreal: Project on Global Working Families, Institute for Health and Social Policy, 2007), www.mcgill.ca/files/ihsp/WFEI2007.pdf, accessed May 8, 2012.

16. Department of Labor, "Family and Medical Leave Act," n.d., www.dol.gov/whd/fmla/, accessed May 8, 2012.

17. Heidi Brown, "U.S. Maternity Leave Benefits Are Still Dismal," *Forbes,* May 4, 2009.

18. Institute for Women's Policy Research, "Maternity Leave in the United States: Paid Parental Leave Is Still Not Standard, Even among the Best U.S. Employers," August 2007, www.genderprinciples.org/resource_files/Maternity_Leave_in_the_United_States_Fact_Sheet.pdf, accessed May 8, 2012.

19. Han, Ruhm, Waldfogel, and Washbrook, "The Timing of Mothers' Employment after Childbirth."

20. Bengt Bjorksten, Lars G. Burman, Peter De Chateau, Bo Fredrikzon, Leif Gothefors, and Olle Hernell, "Collecting and Banking Human Milk: To Heat or Not to Heat?" *British Medical Journal* 281 (September 1980): 765–769.

21. Kathleen Rasmussen and Sheela R. Geraghty, "The Quiet Revolution: Breastfeeding Transformed with the Use of Breast Pumps," *American Journal of Public Health* 101, no. 8 (August 2011): 1356–1359.

22. Maria Makrides, Robert A. Gibson, Andrew J. McPhee, Carmel T. Collins, Peter G. Davis, Lex W. Doyle, Karen Simmer, Paul B. Colditz, Scott Morris, Lisa G. Smithers, Kristyn Willson, and Philip Ryan, "Neurodevelopmental Outcomes of Preterm Infants Fed High-Dose Docosahexaenoic Acid: A Randomized Controlled Trial," *Journal of the American Medical Association* 301, no. 2 (January 14, 2009): 175–182.

23. "Acquired Taste," *New Scientist* no. 2272 (January 6, 2001).

24. Ip, Chung, Raman, Chew, Magula, DeVine, Trikalinos, and Lau, *Breastfeeding and Maternal and Infant Health Outcomes in Developed Countries.*

5. SOUND

1. Alison Gopnik, from comments made during a keynote presentation at the Annual Fall Conference of the Illinois Association for Infant Mental Health in Chicago, October 2, 2009, where the author was in attendance. Dr. Gopnik is author of *The Philosophical Baby* (New York: Farrar, Straus and Giroux, 2009), and, with Andrew N. Meltzoff and Patricia K. Kuhl, coauthor of *The Scientist in the Crib* (New York: Harper Perennial, 2001).

2. W.C. Warren et al., "The Genome of a Songbird," *Nature* 464 (April 1, 2010): 757–762.

3. Dr. Jenny Saffran, interview by author, October 8, 2009.

4. Patricia K. Kuhl, "The Linguistic Genius of Babies," TED Talks, filmed October, 2010, www.ted.com/talks/patricia_kuhl_the_linguistic_genius_of_babies.html, accessed May 8, 2012.

5. P.K. Kuhl, K.A. Williams, F. Lacerda, K.N. Stevens, and B. Lindblom, "Linguistic Experience Alters Phonetic Perception in Infants by 6 Months of Age," *Science* 255 (January 31, 1992): 606–608.

6. Dr. Russell Hamer, interview by author, March 26, 2010.

7. Jenny Saffran, "Words in a Sea of Sounds: The Output of Statistical Learning," *Cognition* 81 (March 2001): 149–169.

8. Lynne Werner, "Babies Have a Different Way of Hearing the World by Listening to All Frequencies Simultaneously," *ScienceDaily* (May 30, 2001).

9. Maria V. Popescu and Daniel B. Polley, "Monaural Deprivation Disrupts Development of Binaural Selectivity in Auditory Midbrain and Cortex," *Neuron* 65, no. 5 (March 11, 2010): 718–731.

10. Dr. Daniel Polley, interview by author, April 29, 2010. All quotes by Dr. Polley in this chapter are from the same interview.

11. A. Kovacs and J. Mehler, "Flexible Learning of Multiple Speech Structures in Bilingual Infants," *Science* 325 (July 31, 2009): 611–612.

12. DiAnne L. Grieser and Patricia Kuhl, "Maternal Speech to Infants in a Tonal Language: Support for Universal Prosodic Features in Motherese," *Developmental Psychology* 24, no. 1 (January 1988): 14–20.

13. Carnegie Mellon University, "Carnegie Mellon Study: Erik Thiessen, 'Adults' Baby Talk Helps Infants Learn to Speak,'" press release, March 15, 2005, www.cmu.edu/PR/releases05/050315_babytalk .html, accessed May 8, 2012.

6. SIGHT

1. Dr. Penny Glass, interview by author, July 15, 2009. All quotes by Dr. Glass in this chapter are from this interview.

2. Dr. T. Rowan Candy, interview by author, November 23, 2009.

3. Penny Glass, "Development of the Visual System and Implications for Early Intervention," *Infants and Young Children* 15 (July 2002): 1–10.

4. Dr. Russell Hamer, interview by author, November 17, 2009. Dr. Hamer is citing the following study: R.L. Fantz, "The Origin of Form Perception," *Scientific American* 204 (1961): 66–72.

5. Beginning in the 1980s, scientists, including Russell D. Hamer, began using visual evoked potential, a new method of studying what infants see. See Hamer, "What Can My Baby See?" n.d., Smith-Kettlewell Eye Research Institute, www.ski.org/Vision/babyvision .html.

6. R.M. Hansen and R.D. Hamer, "The Effect of Light Adaptation on Scotopic Spatial Summation in 10-Week-Old Infants," *Vision Research* 32 (February 1992): 387–392.

7. Dr. Russell Hamer, interview by author, November 17, 2009.

8. Davida Y. Teller, "First Glances: The Vision of Infants: The Friedenwald Lecture," *Investigative Ophthalmology and Visual Science* 38, no. 11 (October 1997): 2183–2203.

9. Dr. Russell Hamer, e-mail correspondence with author, May 31, 2010.

10. Dr. Candy maintains a website with information on infant vision and links to other sites, including an online demonstration of how infants see: www.tinyeyes.com.

11. Hamer, "What Can My Baby See?"

12. Dr. Russell Hamer, interview by author, November 17, 2009.

13. Carla Schatz's section titled "Phoning Home" is within *"How Are the Children?" Report on Early Childhood Development and Learning,* September 1999, U.S. Department of Education, www2.ed.gov/pubs/How_Children?IIEarlychildhood.html, accessed February 22, 2010.

14. D.H. Hubel and T.N. Wiesel, "Receptive Fields of Cells in Striate Cortex of Very Young, Visually Inexperienced Kittens," *Journal of Neurophysiology* 26 (1965): 944–1002. Drs. David Hubel and Torsten Wiesel were awarded a Nobel Prize for this work in 1981.

15. Apoorva Mandavilli, "Visual Neuroscience: Look and Learn," *Nature* 441 (May 2006): 271–272.

16. John T. Bruer, *The Myth of the First Three Years: A New Understanding of Early Brain Development and Lifelong Learning* (New York: Free Press, 1999). Challenging prevailing wisdom, Bruer argues that early brain development is not an all-or-nothing proposition.

17. Dr. Russell Hamer, interview by author, November 17, 2009.

18. Ibid.

19. Dr. Russell Hamer, interview by author, June 7, 2010.

20. Andrew N. Meltzoff and M. Keith Moore, "Imitation of Facial and Manual Gestures by Human Neonates," *Science* 198 (October 1977): 75–78 .

21. Dr. Alison Gopnik, discussion with the author at the Annual Fall Conference of the Illinois Association for Infant Mental Health in Chicago, October 2, 2009.

7. TOUCH

1. K.J.S. Anand and P.R. Hickey, "Pain and Its Effects in the Human Neonate and Fetus," *New England Journal of Medicine* 317, no. 21 (November 1987): 1321–1329.

2. K.J.S. Anand and the International Evidence-Based Group for Neonatal Pain, "Consensus Statement for the Prevention and Management of Pain in the Newborn," *Archives of Pediatric and Adolescent Medicine* 155 (February 2001): 173–180.

3. Ibid.

4. Dr. Alyssa Lebel, interview by author, July 21, 2010. All quotes by Dr. Lebel in this chapter are from this interview.

5. Rita de Cássia Xavier Balda, Ruth Guinsburg, Maria Fernanda Branco de Almeida, Clovis de Araujo Peres, Milton Harumi Miyoshi, and Benjamin Israel Kopelman, "The Recognition of Facial Expression of Pain in Full-Term Newborns by Parents and Health Professionals," *Archives of Pediatrics and Adolescent Medicine* 154 (October 2000): 1009–1016.

6. Aurimery Gomes Chermont, Luis Fabio Magno Falcao, Eduardo Henrique Laurindo de Souza Silva, Rita de Cássia Xavier Balda, and Ruth Guinsburg, "Skin-to-Skin Contact and/or Oral 25% Dextrose for Procedural Pain Relief for Term Newborn Infants," *Pediatrics* 124 (December 1, 2009): e1101–e1107.

7. Liisa Holsti and Ruth E. Grunau, "Considerations for Using Sucrose to Reduce Procedural Pain in Preterm Infants," *Pediatrics* 125 (May 1, 2010): 1042–1047.

8. American Academy of Pediatrics, Task Force on Circumcision, "Circumcision Policy Statement," *Pediatrics* 103 (March 1999): 686–693. For a statement of reaffirmation of this policy, see "AAP Publications Reaffirmed, May 2005: Task Force on Circumcision Policy Statement," *Pediatrics* 116 (September 1, 2005): 796.

9. Anna Taddio, Vibhuti Shah, Cheryl Gilbert-MacLeod, and Joel Katz, "Conditioning and Hyperalgesia in Newborns Exposed to Repeated Heel Lances," *Journal of the American Medical Association* 288, no. 7 (August 21, 2002): 857–861.

10. Anand and Hickey, "Pain and Its Effects in the Human Neonate and Fetus."

11. T.B. Brazelton and J.K. Nugent, *Neonatal Behavioral Assessment Scale,* 3rd ed. (London: Mac Keith Press, 1995).

12. Heidelise Als, "The Newborn Communicates," *Journal of Communication* 27, no. 2 (Spring 1977): 66–73.

13. "Research Says Massage May Help Infants Sleep More, Cry Less and Be Less Stressed," *ScienceDaily* (November 9, 2006).

14. Line S. Loken, Johan Wessberg, India Morrison, Francis McGlone, and Hakan Olausson, "Coding of Pleasant Touch by Unmyelinated Afferents in Humans," *Nature Neuroscience* 12 (April 12, 2009): 547–548.

15. Aniko Korosi, Marya Shanabrough, Shawn McClelland, Zong-Wu Liu, Erzsebet Borok, Xiao-Bing Gao, Tamas L. Horvath, and Tallie Z. Baram, "Early Life Experience Reduces Excitation to Stress-Responsive Hypothalamic Neurons and Reprograms the Expression of Corticotropin-Releasing Hormone," *Journal of Neuroscience* 13 (January 13, 2010): 703–713.

8. PHYSICAL DEVELOPMENT

1. Centers for Disease Control and Prevention, "Assessment of Infant Sleeping Position—Selected States, 1996," *Morbidity and Mortality Weekly Report* 47, no. 41 (October 23, 1998): 873–877.

2. National Institute of Child Health and Human Development, "Back to Sleep Public Education Campaign," updated January 20, 2012, www.nichd.nih.gov/sids/, accessed May 9, 2012.

3. American Academy of Pediatrics, Task Force on Sudden Infant Death Syndrome, "SIDS and Other Sleep-Related Infant Deaths: Expansion of Recommendations for Safe Infant Sleeping Environment," *Pediatrics* 128, no. 5 (November 2011): 1030–1039.

4. J. Mildred, K. Beard, A. Dallwitz, and J. Unwin, "Play Position Is Influenced by Knowledge of SIDS Sleep Position Recommendations," *Journal of Paediatrics and Child Health* 31, no. 6 (December 1995): 499–502.

5. Annette Majnemer and Ronald G. Barr, "Influence of Supine Sleep Positioning on Early Motor Milestone Acquisition," *Developmental Medicine and Child Neurology* 47, no. 6 (February 13, 2007): 370–376.

6. Judy Towne Jennings, quoted in American Physical Therapy Association, "Lack of 'Tummy Time' Leads to Motor Delays in Infants, PTs Say," press release, August 6, 2008, www.apta.org/Media/Releases/Consumer/2008/8/6/, accessed May 9, 2012.

7. Karen J. Bridgewater and Margaret J. Sullivan, "Wakeful Positioning and Movement Control in Young Infants: A Pilot Study," *Australian Journal of Physiotherapy* 45 (1999): 259–266.

8. Dr. Heidelise Als, interview by author, December 7, 2009.

9. C. W. Callahan and C. Sisler, "Use of Seating Devices in Infants Too Young to Sit," *Archives of Pediatric and Adolescent Medicine* 151, no. 3 (March 1997): 233–235.

10. C. T. Myers, H. K. Yuen, and K. F. Walker, "The Use of Infant Seating Devices in Child Care Centers," *American Journal of Occupational Therapy* 60 (September–October 2006): 489–493.

11. Dina Roth Port, "Do Babies Need to Crawl?" *Babytalk* (August 2007): 67–70.

9. STIMULATION

1. Dr. Heidelise Als, interview by author, December 7, 2009.

2. Rebekah A. Richert, Michael B. Robb, Jodi Fender, and Ellen Wartella, "Word Learning from Baby Videos," *Archives of Pediatric and Adolescent Medicine* 164, no. 5 (March 1, 2010): 432–437.

3. Dr. Russell Hamer, interview by author, November 17, 2009.

4. Gilbert Gottlieb, W. Thomas Tomlinson, and Peter L. Radell, "Developmental Intersensory Interference: Premature Visual Experience Suppresses Auditory Learning in Ducklings," *Infant Behavioral Development* 12, no. 1 (January–March 1989): 1–12.

5. Dr. Penny Glass, interview by author, July 15, 2009.

6. Penny Glass, "Development of the Visual System and Implications for Early Intervention," *Infants and Young Children* 15, no. 1 (July 2002): 1–10.

7. "Infant Brain Development," n.d., Mesa Community College website, www.mesacc.edu/dept/d46/psy/dev/Spring99/infant/brain .html, accessed May 9, 2012.

8. Kathleen Kiely Gouley, "Stimulation and Development during Infancy: Tuning In to Your Baby's Cues," n.d., New York University Child Study Center, www.aboutourkids.org/articles/stimulation_ development_during_infancy_tuning_in_your_baby039s_cues, accessed May 9, 2012.

9. Harry T. Chugani, Michael E. Behen, Otto Muzik, Csaba Juhasz, Ferenc Nagy, and Diance C. Chugani, "Local Brain Function Following Early Deprivation: A Study of Postinstitutionalized Romanian Orphans," *Neuroimage* 14, no. 6 (December 2001): 1290–1301.

10. MOM AND DAD

1. Kim Pilyoung, James F. Leckman, Linda C. Mayes, Ruth Feldman, Xin Wang, and James E. Swain, "The Plasticity of Human Maternal Brain: Longitudinal Changes in Brain Anatomy during the Early Postpartum Period," *Behavioral Neuroscience* 124, no. 5 (October 2010): 695–700.

2. Centers for Disease Control and Prevention, "Maternal and Infant Health Research: Pregnancy Complications," revised December 4, 2010, www.cdc.gov/reproductivehealth/maternalinfanthealth/ PregComplications.htm#Depression, accessed May 9, 2012.

3. B.N. Gaynes, N. Gavin, S. Meltzer-Brody, K.N. Lohr, T. Swinson, G. Gartlehners, S. Brody, and W.C. Miller, "Perinatal Depression: Prevalence, Screening Accuracy, and Screening Outcomes Summary," n.d., Agency for Healthcare Research and Quality, www .ahrq.gov/clinic/epcsums/peridepsum.pdf, accessed May 9, 2012.

4. Dean A. Seehusen, Laura-Mae Baldwin, Guy P. Runkle, and Gary Clark, "Are Family Physicians Appropriately Screening

for Postpartum Depression?" *Journal of the American Board of Family Medicine* 18, no. 2 (March–April 2005): 104–112.

5. Cindy-Lee Dennis and Ellen D. Hodnett, "Psychosocial and Psychological Interventions for Treating Postpartum Depression," *Cochrane Database of Systematic Reviews,* 2007, www.health.am/psy/more/psychosocial-and-postpartum-depression/, accessed May 9, 2012.

6. Dr. Aparna Sharma, interview by author, October 29, 2010.

7. Guttmacher Institute, "Requirements for Ultrasound," *State Policies in Brief,* May 1, 2012, www.guttmacher.org/statecenter/spibs/spib_RFU.pdf, accessed May 9, 2012.

8. C.G. Zachariah Boukydis, Marjorie C. Treadwell, Virginia Delaney-Black, Kathleen Boyes, Mary King, Timberly Robinson, and Robert Sokol, "Women's Responses to Ultrasound Examinations during Routine Screens in an Obstetric Clinic," *Journal of Ultrasound Medicine* 25 (February 7, 2006): 721–728.

9. The quotes recorded here are some of the women's responses as Stockman recollected them during an interview by the author, April 16, 2010. All quotes by Stockman in this chapter are from this interview.

10. Ilona S. Yim, Laura M. Glynn, Christine Dunkel Schetter, Calvin J. Hobel, Aleksandra Chicz-DeMet, and Curt Sandman, "Risk of Postpartum Depressive Symptoms with Elevated Corticotropin-Releasing Hormone in Human Pregnancy," *Archives of General Psychiatry* 66, no. 2 (February 2009): 162–169.

11. James F. Paulson and Annie Panno, "Significant Number of Fathers Experience Prenatal, Postpartum Depression," *Journal of the American Medical Association* 303 (May 19, 2010): 1961–1969.

12. Philip Boyce, John T. Condon, Jodi Barton, and Caroline J. Corkindale, "The First-Time Fathers Study: A Prospective Study of the Mental Health and Well-Being of Men during the Transition to Parenthood," *Australian and New Zealand Journal of Psychiatry* 41, no. 9 (September 2007): 718–725.

13. Edward E. Bartlett, "The Effects of Fatherhood on the Health of Men: A Review of the Literature," *Journal of Men's Health and Gender* 1, no. 2 (September 2004): 159–169.

14. E.E. LeMasters, "Parenthood as Crisis," *Marriage and Family Living* 19 (1957): 352–355.

15. Erika Lawrence, Rebecca J. Cobb, Alexia D. Rothman, Michael T. Rothman, and Thomas N. Bradbury, "Marital Satisfaction across the Transition to Parenthood," *Journal of Family Psychology* 22, no. 1 (February 2008): 41–50.

ACKNOWLEDGMENTS

I am indebted to a virtual village of people for their help and support. First of all, the book would not exist without Maureen and Eric Lasher, my agents and good friends. The idea was born over dinner shortly after the birth of the Lashers' grandchild, Anna, and at about the time I welcomed granddaughters Carissa and Molly. Maureen and I watched our daughters as new mothers and remembered our own bewilderment when our children were newborns. What's really going on with an infant during those first three months? we wondered. Maureen said, "There's a book here."

I thank my editor at the University of California Press, Naomi Schneider, for agreeing. She believed in the book from the start. I thank her especially for her suggestions for a succinct and strong introduction. A team of reviewers who read early versions of the book also helped strengthen and polish the ideas.

I believe that professionals who study the brains, behavior, and development of infants do so because they have a love for children that is as deep and as powerful as their love of science. I'm grateful to so many scientists, researchers, and health care providers for explaining their research, showing me their labs, and giving me hours of their time to help me communicate the latest findings in infant research.

I especially thank Dr. James McKenna, Dr. Heidelise Als, Dr. Russell Hamer, Dr. Jennifer Saffran, Dr. Linda Gilkerson, Dr. Penny Glass, the staff at Pathways Awareness in Glenview, Illinois, and the doulas of Birth Journeys in Burlington, Vermont.

The world that real-life families inhabit provided a wealth of information. I thank the dozens of mothers and fathers who let me into their homes to talk about their fears and frustrations and their sweet moments with their newborns. There were so many who shared experiences with me, and I thank especially Jessica Rine, Sandy and Frank LeBan, Courtney and John Bowles, Beth Wheeler, and Eric Kettelhut and his wife, Louisa Elder.

Several people gave generously of their time to read and critique chapters, red pen in hand. Susan Baum and June Davidek, my friends since childhood, were trusted readers for content and sticklers for grammar. My mother, Sophia Brink, who could count two children, six grandchildren, and fifteen great-grandchildren among the infants she loved, read every word with intense pride before her death at age ninety-six.

I thank my brother-in-law, Jim Mondek, for supporting me in the use of a story about my sister Nancy. And I thank my children, Jenny Diaz and Rachel Wheatley, for allowing me to use some of our personal family stories.

Finally, I thank Jack Bush, my partner in life, for his clarity of thought. His interest in my work often led to conversations and ideas that made their way into the pages of this book. Always, I thank him for his encouragement and love.

INDEX

Text: 10.75/15 Janson

Display: Janson MT Pro

Compositor: Toppan Best-set Premedia Limited

Printer: Maple Press